Nursing in the Church

A JCN NURSING FOCUS BOOK

Judith Allen Shelly

Editor

NCF Press
A ministry of Nurses Christian Fellowship®
of the InterVarsity Christian Fellowship®
P.O. Box 7895, Madison, WI 53707-7895
World Wide Web: www.ncf-jcn.org
E-mail: ncf@ivcf.org

NCF Press® is the book-publishing division of Nurses Christian Fellowship of the InterVarsity Christian Fellowship/USA®. In response to God's love, grace and truth: The purpose of Nurses Christian Fellowship/USA is to establish and advance in nursing, within education and practice, witnessing communities of nursing students and nurses who follow Jesus as Savior and Lord: growing in love – for God, God's Word, God's people of every ethnicity and culture and God's purposes in the world. NCF is a member movement of Nurses Christian Fellowship International. For information about local and regional activities, contact NCF at the address, E-mail, or website above.

Cover photograph: Carlos Vergara
Cover design: Kathy Lay Burrows

ISBN 0-9723123-0-7

Printed in the United States of America

Library of Congress Cataloging-in-Publication Data

Shelly, Judith Allen, Editor
Nursing in the Church, A JCN Nursing Focus Book.

p. cm.
Includes bibliographical references.
ISBN 0-9723123-0-7
1. Parish Nursing. 2. Community health – religious aspects. 3. Spiritual care.
I. Shelly, Judith A. II. Title.
RT120.P37 C374 2002
610.73'43-dc21 *Library of Congress Control Number: 2002112633*

NURSING IN THE CHURCH

Judith Allen Shelly, Editor

Part Four: Models of Ministry

Part Five: Spiritual Care

Parish Nursing
Firing the Imagination

Judith Allen Shelly

Eileen's eyes sparkled as she told me that her pastor had asked her to begin a parish nurse ministry in their congregation. "I really don't know much about parish nursing, but I think this is what I want to do with the rest of my nursing career," she began. "Somehow I feel that this is why I became a nurse."

Eileen read everything she could find about parish nursing, interviewed parish nurses in her community and signed up for a basic preparation course. In the meantime, she has set up a well-planned program for her church.

What is it about this burgeoning new specialty that tugs at our hearts and fires our imagination?

The church has a long history in health care. It's taken various forms over the centuries, but interestingly, *nursing* has always been the heart and center of church-based health care. Other religions have their *shamans* and witch doctors, but Christianity is characterized by nurture, care and servanthood. What makes the difference?

Nursing as a public role grew out of the life and teachings of Jesus Christ. Nursing, as a response of faith, calls us to servanthood in the name of Christ. Jesus said, "...whoever wishes to be great among you must be your servant, and whoever wishes to be first among you must be your slave; just as the Son of Man came not to be served but to serve, and to give his life a ransom for many" (Mt 20:26-28).

He elaborated further when he said, "for I was hungry and you gave me food, I was thirsty and you gave me something to drink, I was a stranger and you welcomed me, I was naked and you gave me clothing, I was sick and you took care of me. . . . Truly I tell you, just as you did it to one of the least of these who are members of my family, you did it to me" (Mt 25:35-40).

Most nurses (even many who are not Christians) seem to feel, at the deepest level, that we are responding to Jesus' call when we choose nursing as our life's work. Then we face the reality of profit-driven health care, where increasingly fewer RNs must care for higher numbers of more complicated cases with shorter hospital stays. Today's nurses mourn the loss of the personal patient contact that makes our job rewarding. We worry about what will become of patients when they are discharged while still seriously ill. Nurses take responsibility seriously, so we try to cope, and then pay the price in stress-related illnesses. However, in the process, many nurses today also lose the sense of calling that propelled us into nursing in the first place.

Despite the rebellion against our old handmaiden image and the concept of servanthood, nurses know deep down inside that serving is what nursing is all about. We don't really have a problem with serving, but we *do* care about whom we serve. We want to serve God and those he put in our care. We don't want to serve profit-driven systems. In fact, Jesus made it quite clear that "No one can serve two masters; for a slave will either hate the one and love the other, or be devoted to the one and despise the other. You cannot serve God and wealth" (Mt 6:24).

Too many nurses today find themselves unwillingly serving mammon (wealth), and it grates on their souls.

Parish nursing gives us the opportunity to function the way we initially envisioned nursing. We care for people over the long haul, providing continuity in the context of a personal relationship. We care for the whole person in the context of the family and the faith community. While monitoring physical health, we attend to spiritual and emotional needs as well. We work to bring those in our care into *shalom,* a God-centered wholeness that incorporates health, wellness, welfare, peace, happiness, rest, community and prosperity, not merely physical cure. No one is standing over us demanding increased productivity or cost reductions. We have time to spend with each person and family, knowing that God has *lavished* his grace upon them, so we can too (Eph 1:7-8). No wonder nurses around the world are drawn to parish nursing.

However, even parish nursing is entrusted to sinful human beings. We must walk carefully and prayerfully in this newly restored ministry of the church. As the parish nursing movement matures, we must watch several troublesome trends.

First, we have a tendency to become too comfortable. After jumping out of the stress and disillusionment of secular nursing, working in the church feels like a welcome relief. However, our concern must continue to focus on the poor, the sick and the disenfranchised of society—and most of those people will be beyond the walls of a suburban church.

Second, we are tempted to seek the world's approval. While the American Nurses Association's approval of *The Scope and Standards of Parish Nursing Practice* (1998) gives professional status and accountability to parish nursing, we must remember that we are primarily accountable to God and his church. If the movement toward standardization, credentialing and third-party reimbursement continues to mount, we must watch carefully to see that God's standards are not violated, or that we once again find ourselves serving mammon.

Finally, we must not lose sight of the vision. The current shape of parish nursing has been good for nurses and good for the church; however, it is not the only model of church-based health care. If the goal of our vision is *shalom*, we still have a long way to go. Our calling is not only to comfort the sick, but to bring the healing light of Christ's gospel to those who need the Great Physician (Mt 9:12). The way we go about that will change with the culture and the needs of those we serve. We will probably become more involved with providing physical care. We will need more physical assessment skills as well as theological education and ministry skills. We may end up changing systems or building alternative systems to care for those in need. The needs are great. We will definitely need to move out of our comfort zones.

Parish nursing *should* fire our imagination, for it comes from the heart of Jesus. Let's continue to listen carefully to his voice as he leads us into the next phase of restoring health care to its rightful place in the church.

Originally published in JCN, Summer, 2001

Part One

The Church and Health Care

1

We Have Come This Far by Faith

Judith Allen Shelly

Well, you can't know where you're going unless you know where you've been," a friend informed me when I told her that the next issue of *JCN* would focus on nursing history. She was about the third person who said something to that effect in the previous week, and it reinforced my own conviction that we must know our history to interpret the present and plan for the future. History is more than just recalling trivia from the distant past. Our history provides us with identity, perspective and direction.

Until recently, almost every nursing history recognized the teachings and examples of Jesus Christ as the beginning of nursing's public role. Of course people, especially women, have always cared for one another in the family or tribe. Warriors have been nursed back to health for the nation's sake. But the idea of reaching out to the poor, the weak and the dispossessed was uniquely Christian. In fact, early Roman historians commented that the Christians were stupid to deplete their resources by caring for the dregs of society.

That early Christian commitment to caring did not continue with a stellar record. In fact, as the church became institutionalized and spiritually weak, nursing degenerated as well. In times of spiritual revival, nursing reemerged as a ministry of the church. Modern nursing grew out of such a revival in Northern Europe in the late 19th century.

Nurses have identified with Florence Nightingale for the past hundred years. Nightingale's role model led to professional standards in nursing practice and vastly improved nursing education, but her example also led to the secularization of nursing. Nightingale herself learned her nursing identity from two important Christian models – the Catholic Sisters of Charity in Paris and the Lutheran deaconess school in Kaiserswerth, Germany. She then developed her own concepts of nursing, attempting to maintain the same standards of caring but without the Christian foundation.

During this same period, the revival in Northern Europe and America produced parallel movements, both of which enabled the Nightingale system of nursing education to flourish. Christians became deeply aware of both the physical and spiritual needs of their neighbors and of people in other countries. The deaconess movement in Germany, Holland, England and Scandinavia rapidly burgeoned. Deaconess schools and hospitals spread throughout Europe and North America. At the same time, dozens of mission societies sprang up, sending missionaries around the world to establish schools and hospitals. Many of these hospitals adopted the Nightingale system of nursing education. The two philosophies co-existed quite comfortably for a hundred years because both were also strongly influenced by the spirit of the age – modernism – with its optimistic view of human progress.

Today a new, post-modern spirit influences our age, with shifting identities, perspectives and direction. Recent nursing histories no longer pay much heed to the influence of Jesus Christ but instead hearken back to witches, crones and *shamans*. Were the old history books wrong? Have we gained new knowledge? Not really. Much of this revisionist history has been constructed to explain recent changes in nursing practice and education influenced by the new paradigm. The Christian values of servanthood, commitment and sacrifice no longer feel comfortable to nurses who want autonomy, personal comfort and ethical relativism.

The present health care crisis should not surprise us if we are familiar with nursing history. We have simply come to a fork in the road. For the past hundred years, we have been traveling on a combined interstate highway that ultimately had to split in two directions. Now we have to choose. Will we follow Phoebe (Rom 16:1-2), Fabiola and Hildegard? If so, we may choose a servant role, lower pay, fewer benefits and a life of deep satisfaction. On the other hand, we can follow *shamans*, witches and crones. That may provide power, prestige and financial gain, but we may lose souls.

Right now the insecurity of restructuring, corporate takeovers and vastly changing roles seems overwhelming. But I believe that the current crisis is one of the best gifts God has given the church, and the nursing profession, in a long time. It makes us look at who we are, where we have come from and where we are headed—and forces us to make a choice.

Jesus told his followers in Matthew 6:24, "No one can serve two masters; for a slave will either hate the one and love the other, or be devoted to the one and despise the other. You cannot serve God and wealth."

We have become too comfortable with wealth, and too often lose sight of God. Jesus' disciple, Peter, learned the hard way that taking his eyes off Jesus was a disastrous strategy. In the Gospel story of the disciples being besieged by a storm on the Sea of Galilee, Jesus came to them, walking on the water (Mt 14:22-33), and they were so frightened by the wind and the waves that they did not even recognize Jesus. They thought he was a ghost. Peter, in his cynicism, said, "Lord, if it is you, command me to come to you on the water" (v. 28). He did fine until he took his eyes off Jesus to see the waves and feel the wind. Then he sank.

Nursing feels like a little boat on a stormy sea right now. We can choose to focus on the wind and waves, trying anything we can do just to survive, or we can choose to follow Jesus. He may not lead us where we think we want to go, but I can guarantee that we won't sink—and the destination is glorious.

Originally published in JCN, *Spring, 1997*

2

The Caring Congregation
A Healing Place

Phyllis Ann Solari-Twadell

Today as the "Healthy People 2000" time frame dwindles, and the health care system finds itself in volatile flux, health care leaders are more interested than ever in the role that the church can play in health. They recognize that future improvements in health will come only as people assume greater responsibility for their health and for the health of their communities. As Tom Droege, associate director of the Carter Center Interfaith Health Program, says, "This is a spiritual problem calling for changes in behavior, not a medical problem calling for a scientific breakthrough."[1]

The parish nurse can be a catalyst for individuals and communities of faith to come to this understanding. Parish nursing provides an opportunity for a congregation to exercise its potential to be a health place and community of healing. Through providing whole-person care, the parish nurse models an understanding of health as being more than physical, and stewardship including how people care for their gift of health.

In the *American Journal of Health Promotion*, "Church Based Health Promotion: An Untapped Resource for Women 65 and Older," Lynda Ransdell listed eighteen reasons why church-based health promotion programming is successful.[2] What was interesting, however, was what was missing from this list. No mention was made of the historical, theological foundation that is integral to congregational life and relates directly to health, healing and wholeness.

The gospel and the tradition of the church that affirms that health is life as God intended it to be was absent. The notion that humanity, according to Scripture, is created "in the image of God" (Gen.1:26-27) was missing. The church as the body of Christ called to be a community that chooses life and promotes health in its most comprehensive terms: individual, communal, societal, global and cosmic, was not mentioned.[3] The people of God trusting God, supporting each other, ministering to each other through the Word and sacraments, and caring for one another with all the "goods" God gives, being sustained by individual and common ministries, in the process of healing toward ultimate health, was overlooked.[4]

This theological foundation, which provides a basis for the congregation to assist its members in developing value systems, is an important ingredient in undergirding a healthy life. These value systems fostered through participation in a faith community frequently result in behaviors that contribute and sustain the individual in living a healthy lifestyle, a lifestyle often challenged by a society and culture that perpetuates messages and patterns of living contrary to these religious beliefs and values.

In an emerging faith and health movement, congregations are in a pivotal position to reshape public awareness of health as something more than the absence of disease. Congregations promote health through community building, enhancing the meaning of life, and nurturing core spiritual values, a purpose for living and social justice for the poor and underserved.[5]

What a Congregation Can Do

I use the term *congregation* to mean "an assembly of people whose beliefs about God combine with a common identity, a shared history, regular worship and common values in order to effect personal and social transformation."[6] Although congregations have characteristics common to other human social systems, they are also shaped by values and practices unique to their beliefs and identity. Inherent in this belief and identity is the understanding that congregations are a catalyst for growth and change, and a potential source for health through being a healing and sustaining community. The primary functions of any congregation are teaching, preaching, fellowship, worship, service and advocacy; each has a role in health.

Teaching. At a 1989 conference "Striving for the Fullness of Life: The Church's Challenge in Health," sponsored by the Carter Center in Atlanta, Georgia, and the Wheat Ridge Foundation of Chicago, William Foege, MD, then executive director of the Carter Center, outlined five differences the church can make in health education. Most important was his introductory statement that the church "can provide a larger and more complete vision of health."[7]

Foege's five educational focuses are: 1) the church can teach us about "the unity of body and soul and about the damage caused by the inability to see people as wholes"; 2) the church can teach us about the importance of the unity of people: the responsibility to care for our neighbor; 3) the church can be instrumental in teaching about the "overlap of medicine and religion"; 4) the church should be teaching about prevention; and 5) the church "should be teaching perspective. Health is not an end in itself. It is not the purpose of life, but it helps to serve life's purpose."

The identification of these five areas of education was followed by an important emphasis: that "church communities need to become communities of people who believe they *can*." Congregations who lack the vision of their important role in health will not be able to fulfill it. The first step is for the mindset of congregational members to begin to embrace a new paradigm for their faith community. Once the vision of the congregation as a health place is understood, myriad contributions can be made to maintain or improve the health status of those it serves.

Preaching. Through symbolism and metaphor, the messages of health, healing and wholeness are present in Scripture. What a gift to members of a faith community when these messages are preached regularly! This would offer to each assistance in discerning for themselves how they need to maintain, modify or change their lives to be better stewards of their gift of health. The God whom Jesus discloses does not intend sickness but health. With whatever messages are preached, with whatever models we explain the phenomena of sickness and healing, this affirmation of God's will for human wholeness must be prominent and stand at the center of a theology of healing and health informed by the Gospels.[8]

Worship. Through worship each is invited to actively engage the awareness that the Creator who gave the breath of life continually sustains life. By worshiping and praying together with minds, hearts, spirits and voices, we acknowledge that the Creator of all life is working through the concrete relationships which impact our lives to renew and support us on our individual journeys. As each person through worship becomes open to the Eternal One, personal longings and attentive listening draw the individual into the community of caring.[9] This act of faithfulness sustains health in a holistic way. Participants in the worship experience are bombarded with assurances that they are not alone. They are part of a community that cares. This idea alone enhances health. Isolation is drummed away by the lifting up of many voices.

The music and song that is chosen as part of worship is important. Many hymns speak of the call to health and wholeness. The experience of music and song alone can soothe the soul and relax the mind and body.

All aspects of the worship experience must be considered as to their provision of a health-filled experience for the worship participants.

Fellowship. An early theoretical framework for understanding the relationship between social support and health was elucidated by epidemiologist John Cassell in the mid-1970s. He noted that disrupted social ties affect the body's defense system so that the individual becomes more susceptible to disease. Sir William Osler's statement that "it is much more important to know what sort of patient has the disease than what sort of disease the patient has" emphasizes the value of knowing the patient.[10] Today a growing number of studies support the idea that the "sort of patient who has the disease" is likely to be one who is not immersed in a strong supportive network or who has recently experienced a disruption in his or her traditional sources of social support.[11] Beside weight, blood pressure and laboratory values, an additional indicator of health is the quality of relationships in one's life. Relationships are fostered within the life of a congregation. For many, some of their most significant relationships are developed through congregational involvement.

Service. The highest vision of a faith-filled person is to fulfill a mission of service.[12] Service sits at the foundation of a spiritually oriented life. Being a good steward of one's personal health resources is not only important in terms of insuring good health for the individual as a final goal, but good health becomes a means by which the individual is enabled to serve others. The challenge is to use one's energy and knowledge for self care and, at the same time, be able to reach out to meet the needs of another.

The church provides ample opportunity to serve others through various ministries. The church as a volunteer organization is built on the trust that the community of the faithful will largely exist on the service provided by the members of that community. Through the service provided, the health of the community supports the health of the individual. The health of the individual in service to another supports the corporate health of the congregation.

Advocacy. Congregations interface with the private and public spheres of life. They provide substantial stability to a person's private life by translating for their members the meaning of life and transcendence, as well as by giving them a personal identity and sense of belonging in the community. In the public sphere, churches act as important instruments for conveying the operative values of society, framing the moral dimensions of political questions and aspiring to decipher the biblical message for today's questions. The congregation that serves the external civic community is distinguished by the willingness to: 1) identify problems that put the health of individuals in the community at risk; 2) be in open dialogue about the issues related to those problems; and 3) highlight the socially responsible thing to do for the common good. The congregation as a transmitter of cultural and moral values has a duty to respond when these values are in jeopardy with the society's stance and press for change in the social order.

Advocacy is an important function of a healthy faith community. It stresses the urgency of maintaining a civic environment that perpetuates health and insures that the quality of life will be enhanced in the living environment that surrounds the congregation. Furthermore, it insures for members of the congregation a level of safety and security in their living environment which, in turn, causes less stress and a more harmonious ambiance within the civic community.

Foundations and Framework for Parish Nursing

A concrete expression of their mission of health, for many congregations, is seen through the development of a parish nurse program. Foundations of this ministry are: 1) hope, the reaching out for courage, meaning and wholeness; 2) mutuality, an interacting contribution occurring between a person and the world, or between two people, or between a person and God, from which something new and free is born; 3) faith, the conviction about the not-yet-proven; 4) grace, the mystery of God's intense living presence in us; 5) imagination, the vehicle for hope, necessary to envision what is truly possible; 6) desire, a virtue in that it has determination and refuses to give up easily; 7) patience in waiting, not putting something on the back burner but committing ourselves to the attainment of our dream. This is why we wait.[13]

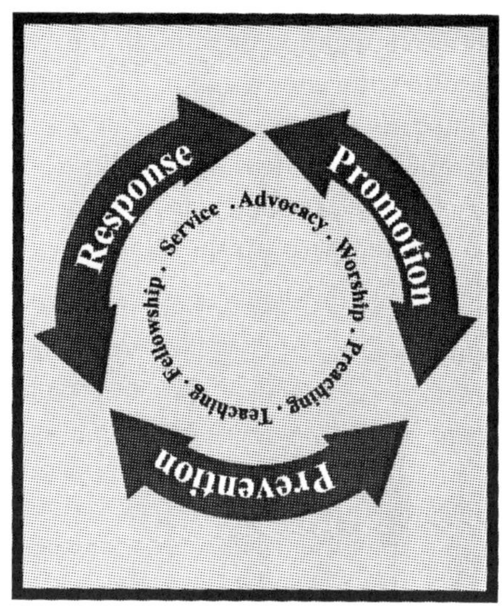

Metropolitan Chicago Synod (1989). Health and Healing for Church and Community, *unpublished manuscript, International Parish Nurse Resource Center, Park Ridge, Illinois.*

Along with this foundation, it is helpful to have a framework in which to begin to define the focus of this ministry. A suggested framework is that of health promotion, prevention and response.

Health promotion focuses on healthy human development rather than response to specific health problems. For example, at a church potluck dinner a congregation's health cabinet may offer one table of foods specifically prepared with healthy recipes. Recipes can be displayed next to the dishes on the table. Those on restricted diets can see what the ingredients are and if they can eat the food. It also offers other members an opportunity to make a knowledgeable choice of what foods they want to eat.

Prevention highlights the lowering of risk factors and reduction of the incidence of illness, including preventing the premature occurrence of chronic illness. Prevention can consist of the basic offering of alternatives and choices for members of the congregation or through the development of support groups. If a congregation has a number of members who are diabetics or arthritics, offering a support group in which the people who have the same illness make contact and get to know each other can reduce feelings of isolation and depression often associated with chronic illness.

Response is the action taken to address actual problems that can affect health and healing. Of these three emphases, response is the most commonly seen in operation within a congregation, with or without a parish nurse structure in place. Providing meals to those who are sick is an example of a response to a crisis that a member may be experiencing.

Important to Lay the Groundwork

It is essential that those interested in developing a parish nurse program in their church spend time assisting the members of the faith community in understanding the theological basis of the congregation as a health place and community of healing. It is only through helping people to gain this mindset that the health mission of the congregation can be vitalized. If this important groundwork is overlooked, people in the church will tend to understand health as primarily physical, and the concept of nurse as being mainly medical.

The true meaning of the whole-person dimension of care provided through this health promotion, disease prevention nursing role will be difficult to understand, and the theological basis of health will be overlooked. Before the kingdom can change, people must change. Take the time to help the people in your church to understand how their thinking needs to change to embrace the gifts of the parish nurse ministry.

Originally published in JCN, Winter, 1997

NOTES

[1] Tom Droege, "Congregations As Communities of Health and Healing," *Interpretation* 49 (1995): 117-29.

[2] Lynda Ransdell, "Church-based Health Promotion: An Untapped Resource for Women 65 and Older," *American Journal of Health Promotion* 9, no. 5 (1995): 333-36.

[3] Ralph Peterson, *A Study of the Healing Church and Its Ministry: The Health Care Apostolate* (New York: Div. for Mission in North American Lutheran Church in America, 1982), p. 13.

[4] Paul Goetting, "The Christian Congregation As a Healing Community," *Health and Healing: Ministry of the Church* (Chicago: Wheat Ridge Foundation, 1980), p. 78.

[5] Herbert Anderson, "The Congregation As a Healing Resource," in *Religious and Ethical Factors in Psychiatric Practice*, D. Browning, T. Jobe and I. Evison, eds. (Chicago: Nelson-Hall, in assoc. with The Park Ridge Center for the Study of Health, Faith and Ethics, 1990), pp. 264-87.

[6] Ibid.

[7] William Foege, "The Vision of the Possible: What Churches Can Do," *Second Opinion: Health, Faith, Ethics* 13, (1990): 36-42.

[8] John Carroll, "Sickness and Healing in the New Testament Gospels," *Interpretation* 49 (1995): 130-42.

[9] Bob Baylor and Lavone Baylor, *When We Pray: A Prayer Journal for Pastors and Worship Leaders* (Cleveland: United Church Press, 1995), p. ix.

[10] John Cassell, "An Epidemiological Perspective of Psychosocial Factors in Disease Etiology," *American Journal of Public Health* 64 (1974): 1040-43.

[11] Meredith Minkler, "The Social Component of Health," *American Journal of Health Promotion* (Fall 1986): 33-38.

[12] John McKnight, *The Careless Society: Community and Its Counterfeits* (New York: Harper Collins, 1995), p. 176.

[13] Granger Westberg, *Theological Roots of Holistic Health Care* (Hinsdale, Ill.: Holistic Health Centers, 1979), pp. 73-90.

3

Reclaiming the Church's Healing Role

Janice M. Striepe

Is the world healthier now than in the first century? I think of sophisticated medical advances such as laser surgery, organ transplants and Hickman catheters. I remember the extraordinary progress in this century brought by improved sanitation, immunizations and other developments.

Then I reflect deeper. Are the same problems that Jesus observed still present in the world? Today I think of AIDS, wars, poverty and homelessness, family difficulties and mental illnesses. I think of the increase in teenage pregnancies, adolescent suicides and the continuing problems of drug and alcohol abuse. Theologians have talked about the dramatic increase of *brokenness* in the world—*broken* persons, families, communities, and even churches.

A woman in a television commercial praises a brand of aspirin declaring, "I don't have time for pain!" Too often, we have wanted a quick fix for pain and suffering. And Americans often have gone to great measures to deny death.

History of Christian Healing

We are aware of the close connection between healing and the early church. Most hospitals were founded by religious orders or denominations. Many nursing homes have religious affiliations.

Nursing also has roots in Christianity. Phoebe, a deaconess in the early church, is often considered to be the first nurse. After becoming a follower of Jesus, this rich woman opened her home to the sick and cared for them (Rom 16:1-2). Deaconesses were the earliest organized group of nurses.

Later, Roman matrons who converted to Christianity established hospitals and dedicated their lives to the needs of the poor. Numerous religious orders of nursing sisters were established during the Middle Ages. Florence Nightingale felt that the nursing role included ministering to the spiritual as well as physical and emotional needs. She also emphasized prevention and service to those in need.

However, over the centuries the distinction between physical and spiritual care has widened. Doctors and nurses tended our bodies, and pastors tended our souls. The words *health* and *healing* became associated with cure, absence of disease and lack of physical pain. We forgot that the original meanings of health and healing are *wholeness*. In Greek, salvation and healing are the same word.

Throughout the Bible we find numerous instructions about health. Healing was a central component in Jesus' earthly ministry. Jesus, the Great Physician, healed people physically, emotionally and spiritually. In fact, accounts of Jesus' healings make up over one-third of the Gospels; in Luke alone there are twenty-four healing stories. The book of Acts is full of accounts of the apostles' healing.

In the first three centuries of Christianity, healing was considered part of the church's ministry. The liturgy was associated with healing, and the Eucharist was used as a redemptive, as well as a healing, liturgy. Oil was offered with the bread and wine and was also used for anointing the sick. Special healing services developed, with oil and the laying on of hands.

In the fifth century, St. Augustine stated that Christians should not expect the gifts of healing to continue, but that occasional healings might occur. So, healing ministries became the exception, rather than the rule.

During the Dark and Middle Ages (A.D. 590-1517), the ministry of healing for physical and mental illnesses lay forgotten. Although monasteries cared for the sick, the church held a negative attitude toward medicine. The church forbade monks to study medicine and barred Christians from performing surgery. Christian healing did continue through the healing miracles of saints.

The Reformation (A.D. 1517-1648) resulted in less interest in healing, and the Renaissance movement (A.D. 1648-1789) completely destroyed Christian healing ministries. Renaissance scholars and historians promoted science and rational thinking and ignored spiritual dimensions.

But then in the 1800s, there was a dramatic change. People began to reclaim healing in the churches. The Pentecostal churches led the way, but soon Christians of many denominations were focusing on healing.

The 20th century brought new developments. For example: William Branham, a Baptist minister, toured the U.S. and Europe in the 1940s with a healing focus; Oral Roberts began his television ministry; Agnes and Edgar Sanford wrote books and started the School of Pastoral Care in the 1950s; Kathryn Kuhlman published her book *I Believe in Miracles* in 1962; Emily Gardner Neal established a ministry of healing in the Episcopal church in the 1960s; Vatican II (1962) opened the door to develop ministries of healing; Francis MacNutt became highly respected for his work in healing in the Roman Catholic church during the 1960s and 1970s.

In the past ten or fifteen years, nurses and pastors have written books and articles about faith, healing, spirituality and holistic health. Interest is increasing in the role of faith as it relates to physical, emotional or spiritual brokenness.

Wounded Healers

You have probably had a major brokenness experience. And during that time, your faith, your church and your Christian friends may have been important in your experience. Perhaps in your suffering you may have wanted an easy, painless solution. I have had those experiences twice.

In September 1966 I began my senior year at Fairview Hospital School of Nursing in Minneapolis. I was so happy. But on Christmas Eve, I wanted a quick fix, and I wanted to deny that I might die in a few months. Five days earlier, I had an emergency colon resection for a malignant tumor. At midnight I was sobbing as I asked God the "big questions": *Why me? What do you want from me? What am I supposed to do with my life? Is there a reason for this? What is it?*

My night nurse walked in, shining her flashlight at the bottom of my bed. She immediately got a chair and sat down next to me. She reached for my hand and quietly listened as I poured out my heart. I ended by saying, "I know I sound terrible. I shouldn't talk like this on Christmas."

She didn't judge me. She gave me a hug and said, "Just remember some of your favorite Bible verses. One of mine is, 'My grace is sufficient for you, for power is made perfect in weakness' (2 Cor. 12:9). It's okay to be weak and human. God's grace is with you."

Her caring made me feel at peace. I was so thankful that she allowed me to talk about Jesus, and that she shared her own faith. I began to realize that suffering can be a blessing. It's our *attitude* about an illness, a loss or any type of suffering that determines if we grow as a person. I began to "let go and let God."

I prayed and meditated on Bible verses, sometimes angrily shouting at God, "Prove your words!" God did. The Holy Spirit comforted and guided me during the months of completing my RN education. After graduating, the doors opened, and I was happy and at peace when I learned that an organization, World Brotherhood Exchange, matched professionals for short-term volunteer work on mission fields. If I was going to die young, I wanted to make a difference.

I spent six memorable months at Yagum Hospital in New Guinea. The primitive hospital was surprisingly holistic. We were short of medicines, hot water and modern equipment, but we were long on love and caring. Family members bathed their ill loved ones; visiting restrictions were nonexistent; long walks outdoors were the norm; and I had time to talk to and listen to patients, their families and nursing students.

One day Sharone, a nursing student at the hospital, said, "I want to be a missionary nurse in America. Do you think that is a good idea?" I gave her a hug, laughed and said, "Yes, most definitely."

Her comment was insightful. Christian churches there have normally sent teams of pastors, doctors and nurses into mission fields. I thought to myself, *Why isn't this done in established churches in America?*

After I returned home in 1967, my life was average. I married a wonderful man, had two children and continued my nursing career and education. Although there were stressful times in balancing marriage, children and nursing, the years passed happily and swiftly.

Then, in the summer of 1984, the second major brokenness event occurred. I suffered burnout. Things happened in my community health job that made me feel ostracized. I was angry at my nursing colleagues for many reasons. Once again I asked God "the big questions." For months I was in an emotional turmoil. Then in December 1984, I met Jan Burg. She had heard Granger Westberg speak and had started parish nursing in her church. I remembered thinking, "My New Guinea friend, Sharone, was right!"

Although I was feeling better, I still had flashes of anger. One night in January, I awakened with excruciating pain in my left eye. Immediately the Bible verse, "Why do you see the speck in your neighbor's eye, but do not notice the log in your own eye?" (Mt 7:3) flashed in my mind. This verse had never been particularly familiar to me, and as I dashed to the bathroom to splash cold water into my eye, I thought, *What do you mean, God?* In my heart I knew the meaning.

At 7 a.m. I drove to the homes of my nursing colleagues and asked for their forgiveness for my anger against them. They all forgave me. I experienced the power of reconciliation.

Parish Nursing

Later that morning I talked to my pastor about parish nursing. He was very supportive, and together we discussed how to begin this new ministry. In the past seven years, I have had many experiences as a parish nurse in a 350-member congregation.

I responded to a call at church from a health care center nurse. "Alma is critical. The family wants a pastor." My response was, "Our interim pastor lives twelve miles away, but I can come over right now." I experienced momentary panic. Then I gathered my thoughts, prayed, collected my Bible and devotional book, left a message at the pastor's house and went to the nursing home.

As I entered the room, six family members were present. After I introduced myself, I went over to Alma. As I talked to her, I assessed her: no response to verbal stimuli, pulse regular and full, breathing rapid but not labored, warm to the touch, no mottling. Death was not imminent. I knew I had time to get acquainted with the family, and I asked them to tell me about Alma.

This proved to be a heartwarming experience. I asked the family to participate in devotions and suggested to her son that he take Alma's right hand and join hands with me, and complete the circle around the bed by holding Alma's left hand. After the prayer, I read a few Bible verses, a short devotion and concluded with a prayer.

I felt the presence of the Holy Spirit that day and learned how comforting the familiar Bible passages are to people. This experience also illustrates the combining of the pastoral and nursing roles—my assessing, use of Scripture, prayer and reminding the family to talk to Alma since, despite lack of response, she could probably hear. I encouraged them to talk with her about their life memories. I remembered that dying people can be *whole;* our wholeness depends on being in harmony with God, ourselves and others.

During a routine visit to a church member in a health care facility, I asked Mary what was the worst part about being there. To my surprise she said, "I really miss having good chili." In the previous month Mary had become weak and depressed. The week following our visit was an extremely busy one for me, but her comment haunted me. So, at 10 p.m. one night I made chili. The next day I called Mary and said that we were going to share a chili dinner in her room that night. We had a delightful time together as we ate and visited.

This experience, like so many others, reinforced two things for me. First, listen to the Holy Spirit. And second, being spiritual is not necessarily *God talk* but any caring act when a specific need is met. I felt that Mary's spirit was nurtured through the food and companionship. Mary died two weeks later.

Another day I visited Josie, a delightful elderly widow who has intermittent bouts of various illnesses, including hypertension. When I checked her blood pressure, the readings were dangerously high. Josie agreed that she needed to see her doctor. I called her physician's nurse, relaying the blood pressure readings, and was instructed to bring her to the office. We were soon ushered into the doctor's examining room.

The physician was pleasant and thorough during the examination and interview. After giving Josie instructions about a new medication and other aspects of her illness, he turned to me and asked, "Could you check her blood pressure tomorrow?" When I said yes, he paused and asked, "Are you a public health nurse?" I answered, "No, I'm a parish nurse." He replied, matter-of-factly but not unkindly, "Oh then you have no official capacity." I chuckled inside.

That evening I replayed the event to my husband and then sarcastically commented, "I guess I have to be part of some health care delivery system to be official." My husband, a hospital administrator and familiar with health care acronyms like PPOs, DRGs and HMOs, paused a few moments, then quipped, "Next time, just say you're with the OHO, the Original Health Organization!"[1]

Whenever I question my parish nurse role or the parish nurse concept, I remind myself of that fact. Yes, I'm part of the OHO. There is no doubt in my mind that parish nurses can provide a viable addition to the ministry of the church and the health care system.

A favorite verse of mine is, "...all things work together for good for those who love God" (Rom 8:28). Yes, *all* things. The joyful events, but also the sad, suffering experiences, help us to become *wounded healers* and allow the living Christ within us to reach out to our brothers and sisters in Christ.

Verna Benner Carson wrote, "The greatest gift the nurse has to give to clients is one's personal, living, spiritual richness. This gift of one's true self, given in care to the client experiencing crisis, will inevitably encourage the client toward spiritual well-being."[2]

Parish nursing is one way to assist the church to reclaim its healing ministry. But each Christian nurse contributes to this renewed ministry. Nurses and pastors are the only professionals who are *there* for the first cry of life to the last sigh of life. What a blessing that is.

Originally published in JCN, Winter, 1993

NOTES

[1] Janice M. Striepe, *Nurses in Churches: A Manual for Developing Parish Nurse Services and Networks* (Park Ridge, Illinois: Parish Nurse Resource Center, 1989), p. iv.

[2] Verna Benner Carson, *Spiritual Dimensions of Nursing Practice* (Philadelphia: W. B. Saunders Company, 1989), p. 21.

4

Parish Nursing
20th Century Fad?

David Zersen

Parish nursing addresses an important need in the lives of Christians, yet many congregations treat it with suspicion. In a society riddled with change, the movement may seem to some as just another fad. Others may question the appropriateness of the role as an expression of ministry within the local church. Some may wonder why nursing responsibilities are not simply left to clinics, or even the community.

A historical perspective on the current parish nurse movement may help Christians to appreciate it, not only as valid within the contemporary church but also as an extension of the church's healing ministry, which has had various expressions throughout the centuries. While Dr. Granger Westberg is rightly acknowledged as the spirit behind the present movement in the U.S., the idea did not come out of the blue.

Christians' holistic needs were addressed in a variety of parish settings over the centuries. Notable among them were early Christian deaconesses, *Gemeindeschwestern* in 19th century Germany, and Episcopal, Methodist and Lutheran sisters of the same period in the U.S. The fact that their stories are often forgotten may give rise to the notion that parish nursing is a fad. Failing to root the current movement in its tradition can impoverish it, both in spirituality and practice.

Remembering the role of women in meeting the physical needs of local Christians in the earliest church provides important historical roots for the contemporary role of the parish nurse. The female deacon (the feminine form *diakonissa* does not appear in the literature until the early fourth century) of early centuries assisted with the anointing of women at baptisms, with postbaptismal instruction and with the general evangelization of women. Deaconesses also had specific responsibilities for meeting the physical needs of women.

The *Didascalia Apostolorum,* dating from the early third century, describes church life in a Jewish-Christian community in Syria or Palestine. It explains the need for attention to physical needs by the female deacon, "for there are houses whither thou canst not send a deacon to the women on account of the heathen (issue of giving offense), but thou mayest send a female deacon . . . for a female deacon is required to go into the houses of the heathen where there are believing women, and to visit those that are sick, and to minister to them in that of which they have need, and to bathe those who have begun to recover from sickness."[1]

Deaconesses Show Christian Caring

Not only is the character of such women of interest, but also their numbers in congregational settings. In Constantinople, for example, a Christian woman named Olympias (born A.D. 368) was widowed after two years of marriage and decided to give herself to service in the church. Ordained as a deaconess while still under thirty, she devoted herself to the poor and sick with such zeal that Chrysostom had to encourage her to practice discrimination and wise stewardship.[2] In the same city several centuries later, it was noted that the great church of St. Sophia had as many as forty deaconesses assigned to it, while smaller local parishes might have only six.[3]

While the role of deaconess had a spotty history in the Western church, we get glimpses of women caring for the physical needs of parishioners. Members of Canoness Institutes, attached to cathedrals and large parish churches, helped not only with the baptisms and postbaptismal instruction of women, but also in caring for the sick.[4]

In both East and West the church accepted the validity of female ministry, primarily to meet the physical needs of women and children, because of the New Testament roots of such a ministry.

While scholars disagree as to the actual offices or roles of women in the New Testament documents,[5] there is no question that both men and women cared for the physical needs of others as a part of the church's ministry. First Timothy 5:9-10 says, for example, that a widow who was "put on the list" (set apart for a specific ministry) should be "well attested for her good works, as one who has brought up children, shown hospitality, washed the saints' feet, helped the afflicted, and devoted herself to doing good in every way."

By the end of the tenth or eleventh centuries the role of the deaconess in the East disappeared because baptism (with which deaconesses were so integrally involved) came to be applied mostly to children. In the West it had never been a dominant form of ministry and disappeared by the sixth century.[6]

Deaconesses and other women (with ill-defined responsibilities in the historical record) who ministered to the poor and sick made sporadic appearances in the Reformation and post-Reformation eras. The rise of the Industrial Revolution in Europe, however, with its rapid displacement of people and incumbent poverty and sickness, challenged church leaders to find new ministries to meet needs.

In Germany, Theodore Fliedner and Wilhelm Löhe founded institutions that prepared deaconesses for a variety of religious and charitable work. Fliedner was influenced by the Roman Catholic Sisters of Charity as well as by the social welfare work being done in the Church of England. The women he trained, beginning in 1836, became either teaching or nursing deaconesses. Although many worked in institutions, some were placed in congregations. Deaconesses were addressed by the title *Schwester* (meaning "sister," the German title for a nurse, deaconess or nun), and, if they worked in a parish (*Gemeinde*), they were known as *Gemeindeschwestern* or parish nurses—and thousands of them in Germany are still known as such today. It is specifically these parish deaconesses, or parish nurses, sent to cooperate with the clergy and parishioners in providing nursing service and general care to the congregation, whom Fliedner considered his greatest contribution to the life of the church. They were, for that matter, the forerunners of the contemporary visiting nurses or family caseworkers.[7]

In Bavaria, Löhe was influenced as much by the large numbers of unmarried women in the society of his day as Fliedner was by the plight of those displaced and impoverished by the Industrial Revolution.

In 1854 Löhe began a movement to train women for useful work both in the church and society.[8] Through the tireless efforts of these two men, the concept of parish nursing, building on New Testament and early-church foundations, reemerged as a caring service to Christians in local congregations.

Developing the spiritual disciplines of the prospective *Gemeindeschwester* was important in both Fliedner's and Löhe's training. Fliedner's program included the *stille halbe Stunde* (quiet half hour), during which students read the Bible, prayed and meditated. A collection of hymns and Bible readings became their *Missal* wherever they went.[9]

Besides regular community worship, Löhe suggested daily private prayer in this pattern: in the morning, a yielding of self to God; in the forenoon, praise and thanksgiving; at 3 p.m. (the hour of Christ's death), preparation for one's own death; and in the evening, self-examination.[10]

The Movement Spreads

From this impetus, deaconess motherhouses sprang up all over Germany. Likewise in England, a variety of sisterhoods and deaconess movements developed. The German expression was repeated in Scandinavia, parts of Africa (now Namibia and Tanzania) and the U.S. The British expression came to be known in parts of Africa, Australia, India, Canada and the U.S. as well.[11]

In 1846 twenty-four-year-old William Passavant visited Fliedner in Kaiserswerth and begged him to provide some deaconesses for a suburb of what is now Pittsburgh. Thus began the American form of what was largely a hospital-based deaconess movement. One sister of the new institution was a type of parish nurse whose responsibility was to visit in the homes of the Lutherans of the city.[12]

In the U.S. throughout the 19th century, a variety of nursing women with different titles served, largely through institutions, in the Lutheran, Methodist Episcopal and Evangelical United Brethren (now United Methodist) churches. The service of individual sisters in local parishes, however, was unknown.[13] In the 20th century, new expressions of the deaconess movement have arisen, sometimes seen as worship or administrative assistants, but seldom as nurses.[14]

As the parish nursing movement gains momentum in the U.S. (and perhaps ultimately throughout the world), it is valuable to remember those in centuries past who have sought to meet the physical and spiritual needs of Christians as an expression of personal witness and service. A parish nurse who knows the movement's historical roots can also help members of a congregation appreciate the commitment to holistic ministry, which is part of the Christian tradition.

It is also worth remembering that the strength of parish nursing, as it reemerged in 19th-century Germany, lay in the spiritual discipline the nurses received as a part of their training and which they practiced in their ministry. In an era in which Christians generally receive all too little spiritual formation through their local congregations, a deeply spiritual and properly educated parish nurse can be a valuable asset to a congregation, not only in meeting physical needs but also in assisting the clergy with spiritual direction.

Originally published in JCN, Spring, 1994

NOTES

[1] Janet Grierson, *The Deaconess* (London: CIO Publishing, 1981), p. 5.

[2] Ibid., p. 11.

[3] Ibid.

[4] Ibid., p. 14.

[5] Aime Georges Martimort, *Deaconesses* (San Francisco: Ignatius Press, 1982), pp. 24-25.

[6] Ibid., pp. 182-83, 217.

[7] Frederick S. Weiser, *Love's Response* (Philadelphia: The Board of Publications of the United Lutheran Church in America, 1962), pp. 50-51.

[8] Jeannine E. Olson, *One Ministry, Many Roles: Deacons and Deaconesses Throughout the Centuries* (St. Louis: Concordia, 1992), pp. 201-3, 213-15.

[9] Ibid.

[10] Ibid.

[11] Grierson, *The Deaconess*, pp. 97-109; Ludy Rider Meyer, *Deaconesses: Biblical, Early Church, European, American* (Chicago: The Message Publishing Co., 1889), p. 37.

[12] Weiser, *Love's Response*, p. 53.

[13] Olson, *One Ministry, Many Roles*, p. 300.

[14] Ibid., p. 355.

5

What Should the Church Do About Health?

Frances D. Atkins

How do parish nurses make a difference in healing and health promotion in congregations? My study of one church without a parish nurse prompted comparisons with churches that have them.

Health care services are changing rapidly. Third-party payers are providing increasingly limited coverage. Greater numbers of people have little or no health care coverage. Increased demand for health care in the presence of limited resources suggests the need to identify and enhance existing resources that support healing and health promotion. Some government agencies and ministers have identified the church congregation as a healing community engaged in keeping people well. Yet little is known about the views of church members toward their church's role as a healing community, keeping people well or the variety of ways that healing and health promotion occur.

The church for this study serves approximately 500 members in a west central Missouri city of less than 5,000. The city is surrounded by farms in a county that made the transition from being just outside a metropolitan area in the 1980 census to being just inside a metropolitan area in 1990. The church, as old as the city, boasts a prominent location.

The twenty-three church members who participated in the study explored with me their experiences and thoughts about healing and health promotion in their church. Fourteen (61%) were female; nine (39%) were male, with ages from twenty-eight to sixty-seven (mean, median and mode were 44 years). Most were of German ancestry; some were descendants of founding members.

Information came from two audiotaped group interviews during Sunday-school classes, two audiotaped interviews with individual leaders during weekday business hours, and church records. The participants affirmed that their experiences in this church supported healing and health promotion. Several themes emerged from the details given in interviews: a) specific examples of healing and health promotion, b) activities that promote healing and health promotion, c) origin of healing and health promoting activities, d) role of the church in healing and health promotion, e) barriers to the church being a healing community, and f) examples of hurt and pain that are opportunities for healing and health promotion.

Examples of Healing and Health Promotion

Attending church on Sunday helped "things go right the rest of the week" and "wellness inside . . . sanctity . . . peace." Church worship helped one be mentally and spiritually healthy, which in turn led to physical health. Mental health occurred because it "lifts me and changes my perspective," and "you can let down your guard . . . talk about issues that it's awful hard to talk about the rest of the week."

Spiritual teaching helped one person relax, kept another aware of and close to God, thinking about faith in a journey that never ends, seeking what is expected of him in life and wanting to change with strength to change. Emotions were healed through friendships. Church experiences influenced end-of-life decisions for "quality over quantity of life" and "removed fear of death." Health wisdom was learned from others in the church community. Sermons helped give meaning to personal life decisions.

Activities to Promote Healing and Health Promotion

The church setting provided friendships across age groups and "a most important support system." When friends cared, they called and encouraged, gave support during grief, took food and visited, shared in helping others, looked out for each other and provided a safety watch for suicide prevention. Friends helped in "healing your emotions."

One said, "I feel better when friends care." Another said, "After he prayed . . . [I] really started coming out of the anesthetic and being with it." Members gained from visiting the ill at home: "They give so much back to me, more than I give to them." Problems experienced by one helped another: "I knew he understood the situation because he had been there. He gave me a lot of comfort because I knew he understood fully." A visitor after a death helped by his "presence . . . timing . . . shared feelings." Another said, "Support takes care of physical concerns during the ups and downs of life."

Characteristics that helped church members support healing for one another were trustworthiness, loyalty, openness, sharing, consistency, genuineness, honesty, acceptance, being a role model without judging or telling others what to do, loving concern, refraining from gossip or double standards. In addition, everyone had to take part and do something, while realizing their dependence on each other. Mediator skills soothed conflicts between people with different ideas and values. Patience led one to slow down to the pace that another could follow.

Origin of Healing and Health Promotion Activities

Helping one another arose from tradition in the early church. If someone missed church, another went to find out why, and word of mouth spread the need for help. In today's church, need was also the basis for spontaneous and planned responses to help others. Being part of a healing community led one to offer healing ministry.

Activities and programs that contributed to healing and health were preschool classes during the week, support of a shelter for abused children, food and clothing pantries, Weigh Down classes, quilting circles, a crisis support group during the Gulf War, Sunday-school classes, Discovery Groups, Youth on Mission, choirs (adult, youth, handbell), sermons, organized visiting program for homebound members and church camp. A rose on the altar recognized a new birth; a yellow rose marked the absence of a member in the military; a bouquet honored a wedding anniversary.

Role of the Church

Members' expectations of the church suggested their view of the church's role. They expected the church to provide guidance, comfort, help and support where needed. Members realized they were the church: the ones to help provide for each other's needs. They deferred to the pastor for the really tough situations: "When things get threatening, we think he's the only one who can do that."

Some members saw an expansion to a larger role in the future. One said, "It's time for the church to take care of the local community. We've delegated that role to the government, and we need to take it back. The church could do a better job of keeping people well and be much more efficient at it. Some churches are real involved like that. Some of us that are a little more affluent could help. The church needs to be ready to jump in and take over where a bunch of people fall through the cracks. We could help." Peers supported these comments.

Leaders purposefully provided an environment for healing and health. Phrases like "create the desire to participate . . . challenge people to stretch and grow . . . provide a place for things to happen . . . help the youth grow spiritually and mentally through mentoring" described efforts for a healing, healthful place. Sermons and teaching inspired and ministered to members. A variety of worship themes were planned to meet members' needs, while specific world events that touched everyone guided the theme on some occasions.

The teaching ministry was shared by leadership with members. For example, in confirmation classes an adult was paired with each young person for weekly mentoring and teaching, with everyone meeting together monthly for teaching by the pastor.

Administrative leadership provided the structure to manage the healthful environment. A monthly newsletter kept members informed of the many church activities. Volunteer committees divided the work of running this large organization. Additional volunteers carried out the work of the committees. For example, volunteers pledged to visit homebound persons monthly, report to the volunteer committee that organized the visiting, and report to the pastor if the visitor found more than he or she could handle.

Youth on Mission helped needy families with donated work and materials to repair their homes, mow grass or wash windows. Youth on Mission engaged many church members to support youth activities financially, to be trip chaperones, and to welcome the youth in their coming-home reports of where they went, who they helped in what way, and what that meant to both the recipient of the help and to the youth.

Barriers to the Church Being a Healing Community

Despite commitment to their church, members admitted that sometimes it was hard to be a healing community, to share and give when they felt inadequate, criticized, judged or hurt themselves. A need for privacy interfered with openness and sharing. They experienced many demands from work, family and church for their time. Material priorities conflicted with church priorities. Family and church members were sometimes less available to each other since they were pulled in different directions. Some honestly said they "make excuses for not doing something."

The church was no longer the center for socialization. Limited options within the church competed with multiple entertainment options outside the church, both locally and in the nearby metropolitan area. The people with whom members socialized were not necessarily the people at church. Within the church there were so many committees that a member may not know what was going on and, consequently, could lose sight of what was really important.

After being in this church several years, one member said, "We just haven't connected up here yet." City and county characteristics were viewed as obstacles. The comment "too competitive and self-sufficient, with less urgent needs, because the people are not as poor as in other counties" suggested that more urgent needs made it easier to be a healing and health promoting church community.

Opportunities for Healing and Health Promotion

Leaders and members identified the presence of unmet needs. Priorities were given to ministering to families when a member died, visiting the sick, dying and homebound, and tending to the needs of the youth. While activities and programs were already in place, members perceived that more needed to be done in these areas. Ministry for singles, especially for middle-aged, newly single persons, was missing and seen as an unmet need. Impending government welfare budget cuts were viewed as a potential opportunity for the church to move into the community to help those left out of government support.

Conflicts and hurt are inherent among any group of people trying to live out a mission together, and this congregation was no different. Hurt shared within a group attested to the presence of a healing, caring environment, as the group listened and offered their caring. Other situations of hurt shared privately carried the companion message of support and healing that followed the hurt. Some were in the midst of working through the pain in an open, searching journey. All gave opportunities to live out the mission of caring.

Where Do We Go from Here?

The participants in this study reported that they received spiritual, mental, emotional and physical healing from this church community. Many activities contributed to healing and health promotion: support through friendships, inspiration from sermons and teaching, a structured visitation program, Youth on Mission, preschool classes, food and clothing pantry, quilting circles and support for a shelter for abused children. Members saw themselves as the church; therefore, they shared responsibility for the healthful environment.

While many efforts supported healing, members thought more needed to be done among their members and in the broader community. Special concerns were grieving families, the sick and dying, and youth. Some admitted they were unwilling to do more; others were open to more involvement. The history of this church suggested they could accomplish whatever they committed to doing.

In this case study, the activities given high priority were church attendance, support through friendships and a visitation program. The addition of a parish nurse to the ministry team would potentially enhance healing and health promotion by the addition of professional health counseling and screening, locating community resources, giving assistance with referrals and member advocacy, health teaching, volunteer training and facilitation of support groups.[1] While not a common service, occasionally "hands on" nursing care is provided. The amount of time given in service and whether the parish nurse is paid would have an influence on the number and types of activities provided in the congregation.

This comparison of activities in a church without a parish nurse and what churches with a parish nurse on the staff tend to offer suggests that healing and health promotion in a church would be enhanced by the presence of a parish nurse. The next step is to replicate the case study in other denominations to look for consistency of results. Further study would be to follow the change that occurs after a parish nurse is added to a church's ministry team.

Originally published in JCN, Winter, 1997

NOTES

1 Mary McDermott and Joan Burke, "When the Population Is a Congregation: The Emerging Role of the Parish Nurse," *Journal of Community Health Nursing* 10, no. 3 (1993): 179-90.

Part Two

What Is Parish Nursing?

6

Working Toward Shalom

Judith Allen Shelly

Susan stood on my doorstep, a glowing picture of health. Her eyes flashed with enthusiasm for life, and a deep sense of joy radiated from her face. The large mass on her neck betrayed another force at work in her body. Susan was on her way home from radiation therapy for rapidly growing thyroid cancer, but she had never felt more alive.

As a young woman, Susan had a close relationship with God and her church, but something snapped during a serious disagreement with her pastor. Susan grew angry and bitter toward God and the church. She and her husband refused to attend worship, withdrawing from the Christian community.

Her husband returned several years later, and for years the church prayed with him that Susan would release her bitterness and return to church with him. She slipped in occasionally but kept her distance. Then tragedies began to strike. First a son died in an automobile accident. Then Susan's brother died of cancer. Within months Susan faced the same diagnosis.

Throughout all the crises, the church ministered to Susan through notes, visits, flowers and prayers. Susan's thick wall of resistance broke down. She came back to the Lord and into joyous fellowship with the Christian community. But even though Susan was dying, she was alive and well.

What is health? The popular media portray it as youthful appearance, hard muscles, sleek bodies, clear skin and cavity-free teeth. Nursing literature is increasingly moving to the other extreme. Health is "expanding consciousness" according to nursing theorist Margaret Newman.[1] It is "essentially synonymous with becoming, which is an open, rhythmically coconstituting process of the human-universe interrelationship" according to theorist Rosemarie Parse.[2]

Current nursing literature portrays health as a broad concept, so broad, in fact, that it ceases to be an adequate goal for nursing. Newman even states that "health encompasses conditions that heretofore were described as illness, or in medical terms, pathology."[3] For the most part, contemporary nursing's definitions of health focus primarily on a state of mind. Older definitions and conventional wisdom (as represented by television commercials) focus on the body. The World Health Organization (WHO) idealistically defined health in 1946 as "a state of complete physical, mental and social well-being and not merely the absence of disease or infirmity." It was a definition that medical ethicist Daniel Callahan says set the stage for a conception of health that literally encompasses every element of human happiness.[4]

I said that my friend Susan radiated health, despite her tumor. She obviously did not meet the WHO standard of health. On what basis could I say that Susan was "healthy?" What is the difference between that understanding of health and Newman's?

Susan demonstrated health in her attitudes and relationships, but the tumor itself was not encompassed in her health—it remained a serious pathology. However, if we view the person as an integrated whole, created to live in harmony with God, self, others and the environment,[5] then health means being able to function as God created us to be. It involves reconciliation with God and others, forgiving and accepting forgiveness, loving and being loved, finding meaning and purpose in life leading to a sense of joy and hope, as well as freedom from physical ailments.

The biblical understanding of health is closely related to the concept of *shalom*. Often translated as *peace, shalom* actually incorporates all the elements that go into making a God-centered community: peace, prosperity, rest, safety, security, justice, happiness, health, welfare and wholeness. Christian philosopher Nicholas Woltersdorff defines *shalom* as "the human being dwelling at peace in all his or her relationships: with God, with self, with fellows, with nature."[6]

The new Jerusalem described in Revelation 21:2-4 illustrates the meaning of *shalom*. "And I saw the holy city, the new Jerusalem, coming down out of heaven from God, prepared as a bride adorned for her husband. And I heard a loud voice from the throne saying, 'See, the home of God is among mortals. He will dwell with them as their God; they will be his peoples, and God himself will be with them; he will wipe every tear from their eyes. Death will be no more; mourning and crying and pain will be no more, for the first things have passed away.'"

When Jesus cleansed the ten lepers in Luke 17:11-19, only one returned to thank him. Jesus told that man, "Your faith has made you well." All ten were cleansed of leprosy, but only the one who returned found complete healing. The whole point of Jesus healing people was to restore them to a fuller, richer relationship with God.

Let's go back to Susan, my radiantly healthy, dying friend. I visited her as a volunteer parish nurse. We discussed the importance of taking her pain medication and why she didn't have to worry about becoming addicted. We developed a strategy to deal with the side effects. Our primary focus, though, was on her relationships: with her husband, her family, the church community and God. We prayed together, wept and hugged.

As a nurse, I acknowledged the value of expert scientific medical care and also represented the caring Christian community. The role of a parish nurse is somewhere within both. As we combine the best of scientific medicine with the heart of the gospel of Jesus Christ, we work toward *shalom*—a health that draws us into relationship with God and his people and enables us to function as he created us to be.

Originally published in JCN, *Winter, 1997*

NOTES

1 DeAnn Hensley et al., "Margaret A. Newman: Model of Health," in *Nursing Theorists and Their Work,* Ann Marriner, ed. (St. Louis: C. V. Mosby Co., 1986), p. 371.

2 Rosemarie Parse, *The Human Becoming Theory in Practice and Research* (New York: National League for Nursing Press, 1995), p. 13.

3 Hensley et al., "Margaret A. Newman," p. 371.

4 Daniel Callahan, "The WHO Definition of 'Health'," *Hastings Center Studies* 1, no. 3 (1973), 77-87.

5 Adapted from *Spiritual Care: The Nurse's Role,* Judith Shelly and Sharon Fish (Downers Grove, Ill.: InterVarsity Press, 1988), p. 33.

6 Nicholas Woltersdorff, "For Justice in *Shalom,*" in *From Christ to the World: Introductory Readings in Christian Ethics,* Wayne Bouton, Thomas Kennedy and Allen Verhey, eds. (Grand Rapids: Eerdmans, 1994), p. 251.

7

Church Nurse
Caring for a Congregation

Carol J. Smucker

"You're a nurse, so I can tell *you*," began Clara as she opened another dresser drawer. Inside were the disposable pads she used for slight urinary incontinence. She explained the problem. I assured her that it was quite common in women her age and described the exercises she could do to help alleviate the difficulty. Then she showed me around the rest of her "home," a single room in the residence for elderly women.

When our friendly chat was over we prayed together, and she walked me to the door. I gave her a hug, and she waved goodby, promising to recite a favorite poem for me when I came the next time.

Visiting Clara and offering her some friendship and advice are some of the joys of being a health minister. That's the position I've held since completing my master's degree in nursing.

While I was in graduate school, I became more interested in health education. I could envision using my nursing skills in church ministry, visiting the sick and educating the healthy. So, when I saw an ad in a local paper for a health minister in a Lutheran church, I applied. Zion Lutheran Church, a 600-member congregation in Davenport, Iowa, hired me.

Through the Minister of Health Education Program at Iowa Lutheran Hospital in Des Moines, I gained a greater vision for health care ministry in local churches and communities. Along with six other nurses in my class, I learned how to combine nursing knowledge with pastoral care, tuning in to people's spiritual needs, along with their physical and emotional problems. I improved my listening skills and learned how to talk to patients about spiritual matters.

My work at Zion is part of a cooperative program cosponsored by a charitable foundation and the Evangelical Lutheran Church of America. These organizations share the cost of the ministry with the local church for the first three years. In addition to working with the congregation, I spend part of my time ministering to the inner-city neighborhood surrounding the church.

My formal education lasted a year and included weekly classes and time to share experiences with other nurses working in churches. After that program ended, I began meeting regularly with an advisory committee from Zion Lutheran Church that helps me establish goals for my ministry and evaluate my progress.

More and more churches these days are rediscovering their need to take on Christ's ministry of healing. As a health minister, I teach people ways to take care of themselves; aid them in finding the help they need to do that (through resources like medical professionals, support groups or Bible studies); give them health information through screening clinics, educational bulletin boards, newsletters and items in the

Sunday bulletin; and show people how bodies and spirits interact to affect overall health.

At our church we have come to view health not just in terms of physical wellness, but as becoming all a person can be in mind, body and spirit—living for the glory of God. Health is not just an end in itself. It is a process that enhances people's ministry to others by helping them identify their spiritual gifts, giving them training to use those gifts, and building a better sense of fellowship within the congregation.

Unlike hospital work, my job in the church allows me to form long-lasting relationships with people. I met Ted and his wife early in my ministry. At that time Ted was at home, where his wife had cared for him almost ten years. A degenerative muscle disease was gradually robbing him of his independence. Now he is in a nursing home because his wife could no longer care for him.

On a recent visit to the nursing home, Ted met me at the door to his room, grinning widely and clutching the controls of a new electric wheelchair. He talked excitedly about his increased freedom as I walked beside him to the dining room. Many times my ministry consists more in *being* than *doing*—being there to see Ted's new set of wheels.

Much of my time is spent visiting people like Ted. That's where my duties as nurse and minister are inextricably linked. At other times I perform tasks more typical of a nurse. For example, with the help of other nurses in the church, I offer regular blood-pressure screenings. Almost half of the congregation have had their blood pressure checked on Sunday morning. As a result, a number of people have seen their doctors to get treatment. Some have started taking antihypertensive medication; others have changed their diets and lifestyles to lower their pressure.

I offer the same blood-pressure screening service to the community. I set up a table with literature in a local grocery store and check blood pressures at no cost. My card table is strewn with health care literature, and I'm there to talk to anyone who wants to. Some people will talk to me before they'll go to a doctor because there are no strings attached to my services. I believe this is a clear way of showing Christian love to our neighbors in the community.

When I see people seeking help for physical problems, or changing unhealthy lifestyles, or caring for someone else in a new way, or using a newly identified spiritual gift, I know that my ministry is valuable. Recently I felt pleased by the comments that followed a six-week series for people caring for elderly relatives.

"I learned how to talk about the problems I face," one man said.

"I found out that other people have the same problems I do," a woman reported.

"I finally admitted that I had to get help to care for Mother," said another woman.

When this support group for caregivers began, many of the people who came were in crisis situations. They felt unable to cope any longer with the care their family members required. In the group they found insights that helped them to care for themselves and shared deeply with others who were in the same situation they were.

I think one reason these people were willing to come to this support group was because it was led by a nurse. People know that I'm aware of what it takes to care for a sick person. Recently Bill came to me to discuss his chemotherapy. In talking about the treatments, he said, "Well, you're a nurse, so you understand." He was obviously grateful to be able to speak to someone who was both a minister and a person well acquainted with the many side effects of chemotherapy.

Being a health minister means many things. It means being a nurse involved in the healing ministry of the church. And most of all, it means sharing both the highs and lows with people, being there when they are brought down by illness and when they are excited about recovery, walking with them through the ecstasy of childbirth and the grief of death. Being a health minister means sharing in people's lives.

Originally published in JCN, Winter, 1989

8

A Profile of Parish Nurses

Janet K. Kuhn

Parish nursing is an emerging area of specialized nursing. In essence, nurses who choose to practice in this role are those who believe in holistic health, especially focusing on the spiritual dimension as a vital part of health. Their primary emphasis is disease prevention and health promotion, not "hands on" care of clients who are ill.

Currently four models of parish nursing predominate: congregation-based volunteer (CBV); congregation-based paid (CBP); institution-based paid (IBP); and institution-based volunteer (IBV). The models sometimes are combined. For example, a nurse may work in one or more faith communities but be paid a salary and given benefits by an institution.

Employing institutions are most often hospitals but also may be a long-term care facility or a community health agency. When the nurse is employed by a faith community (CBP), the church provides parish nursing services to its parishioners and assumes the salary, expenses and benefits of the nurse. Most parish nurses are employed part-time and work in faith communities.[1]

While specific functions of the parish nurse are determined by the character and needs of the individual institutions or congregations, roles include health educator, health counselor, referral source and coordinator of volunteers and support groups. Another role, particularly in the congregation-based models, is to increase the congregation's awareness of the relationship between faith and health.[2]

Background of Parish Nursing

The first parish nurse program began in 1984 in the Midwest [3] and did not, until fairly recently, appear in the literature. Authors who have written about this new role for nurses have focused on the history of the movement [4] and how to initiate the role.[5] Several have examined parish nursing from a community health perspective,[6] with two authors concluding that parish nursing is an excellent way to extend health care to urban African Americans.[7] Sandra Bergquist and Judith King suggested a framework for organizing the concept of parish nursing, using five broad categories: the client, health, the nurse, the environment and the nursing process.[8]

Research articles are few; however, a descriptive study conducted by Mary Ann McDermott and Joan Burke found that 69 percent of the 109 parish nurses surveyed were between the ages of 35 and 54, and all but one was female. Over half (58%) were salaried, either by a faith community or an institution. Predominant satisfactions with the role were personal and spiritual growth, the ability to practice holistically and the opportunity to establish long-term relationships with clients. Frustrations included unrealistic expectations in the allotted time, ambiguity of the role and its boundaries, and lack of resources, including financial compensation and support systems.[9]

My study was patterned after the previously described one but was conducted in the Northeast. In addition, this descriptive study included interviews, a look at the parish nurse's educational needs and open-ended questions about the role of spirituality in the parish nurse's practice. The purposes were to compare responses to the McDermott-Burke study and to examine perceived education needs of this group.

My Study Methods

The convenience sample was obtained from a list of parish nurses in Pennsylvania in August 1995 supplied by the National Parish Nurse Resource Center and a list of attendees at a two-day workshop in northeastern Pennsylvania. One hundred and twenty-eight questionnaires were mailed with a response rate of 59 percent. Many respondents (36%) were not active parish nurses, so only 48 (N=48) were analyzed. Interviews using the same questionnaire were also conducted with five active parish nurses to obtain more in-depth responses and to confirm the mailed survey findings. Interviewees included two CBP, two CBV and one IBP parish nurses. The institution was a hospital and, interestingly, the nurse worked out of the chaplaincy department, not the department of nursing. The hospital had received a grant to pay her. Two parish nurses worked in a large city, one in a wealthy suburban area and one in a rural community.

The survey questions were based on the published literature and questions I developed. Content validity and clarity were supported by a panel of four experts.

My Findings

The vast majority of subjects (N=47) are women (97.9%), fifty years and older (73%) who received their basic nursing education in a diploma school (62%). Twenty-seven percent were educated in an associate degree program, only 12 percent in baccalaureate programs. Unlike some areas, Pennsylvania has a large number of diploma schools.

Seventy-five percent were CBVs, with 12.5 percent CBP and 12.5 percent IBP nurses. None of the respondents were IBVs. When the nurses were paid, they received a salary ranging from $10-$18 per hour. Part-time employment was the norm (85%). Several indicated they had begun as volunteers and after the first year, they became paid employees.

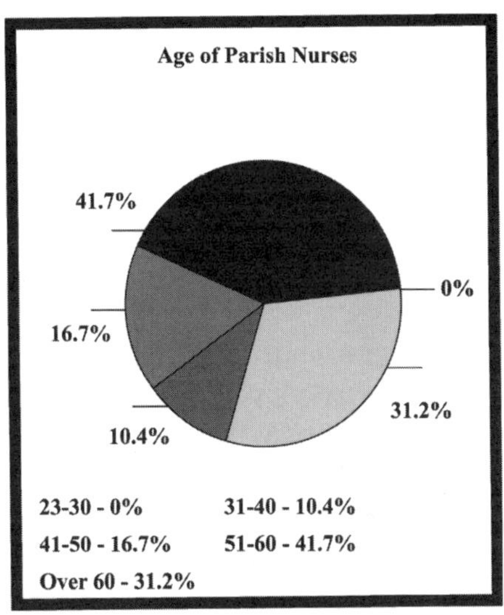

Since titles are often descriptive of our roles, the nurses were asked to indicate what their title was. Most (58%) were called parish nurses, but other titles included health ministries coordinator, health and wholeness team coordinator, health promoter, parish nurse educator and nurse in congregation. Specific professional liability insurance for the parish nurse was maintained by 46 percent of these active parish nurses. Of the 46 percent, 40 percent stated their coverage was paid by their employer. Over half of the remaining respondents have some coverage; however, it was not specific to the parish nurse role.

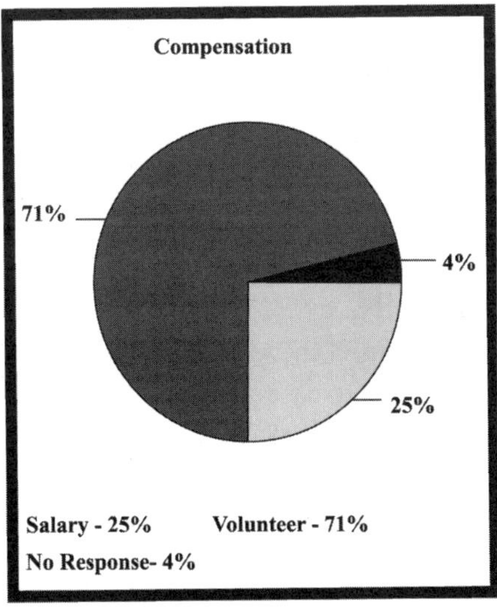

In assessing methods of evaluation of the nurses, 25 percent did not respond to the question, and 25 percent indicated there was no formal process was in place. The remaining 50 percent were formally evaluated quarterly or annually. The basis of evaluation for that 50 percent consisted of reports examining whether personal or employer goals were met, the number of clients visited and the number of educational programs presented. Two respondents commented that they had a verbal evaluation at "random times."

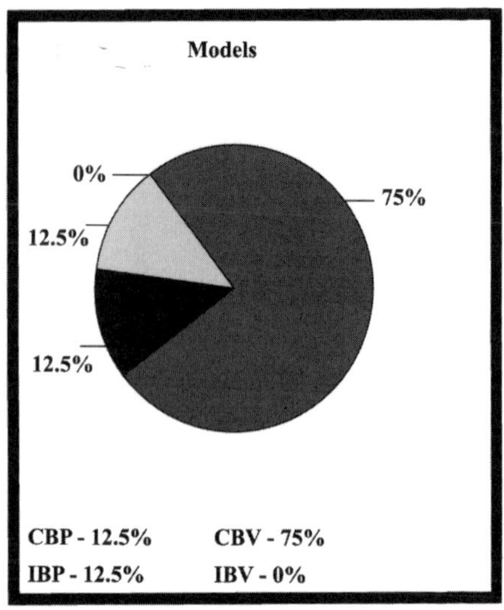

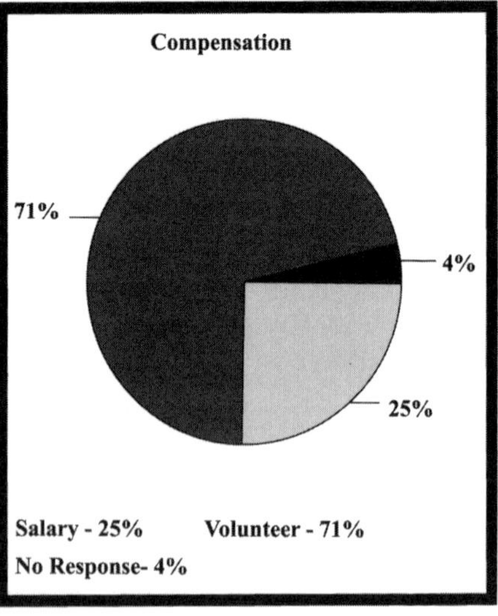

All respondents answered open-ended questions related to the frustrations and satisfactions of this role. Frustrations seemed to be grouped into categories related to too little time, feelings of isolation and the need for support networks, too little money for a salary or resources, and mixed expectations from the clergy and congregation. The satisfactions in the role were reported as the freedom to speak of God and the role of spirituality in health and illness, the "whole ball of wax come into play: body, mind and spirit," developing and maintaining relationships with clients, being an advocate "especially for the elderly," and being a health educator.

Since the intentional incorporation of the spiritual dimension is an integral component of parish nursing practice, nurses were asked to describe how they incorporated spirituality into their role. Comments included: "pray with clients when it seems right," "take Communion to clients," "by promoting wellness of body, mind and soul," "show compassion and caring for all," "offering Care Notes (from Parish Nurse Center)," "frequent discussions as to client's spiritual concerns of family and themselves during illness and terminal diseases," "ask appropriate questions that would give openings for client to respond," "healing service once a month as part of church services," "not going in as a preacher but asking what they want and about their image of the world, following what I hear with what is appropriate to release their pain of spirit," "I formed a Sunday-school class to delve deeper into theological aspects of health and wholeness," "a caring attitude," "emphasizing the worth of every individual," "they know I come through the community of the church," "*just being there* for people," "trying to get a feel for the culture of the community," "sharing Scripture with encouragement."

Additional educational preparation for this role was considered important by 62 percent of the respondents. The subject areas listed included physical assessment skills, especially with the geriatric client, counseling in general and in relation to grief and loss in particular, spiritual assessment, interviewing skills, small-group facilitation, home safety assessment, listening skills, and updates on diagnostic procedures and the treatment of chronic diseases, including patients with AIDS.

My study was necessarily limited by sample size and convenience sample technique. The findings complement those of McDermott and Burke and can be useful to any nurse planning to initiate the parish nurse role. It should be helpful for nurses working with the elderly to become familiar with the role and how these parish nurses function in their geographical areas.

Originally published in JCN, Winter, 1997

NOTES

1 Mary McDermott and Erin Mullins, "Profile of a Young Movement," *Journal of Christian Nursing* 6, no. 1 (Winter 1989): 29-30; Janice Striepe, "The Developing Practice of the Parish Nurse: a Rural Experience," in *Parish Nursing: the Developing Practice* (Park Ridge, Ill.: Parish Nurse Resource Center, 1990).

2 Jean King, Jean Lakin and Janice Striepe, "Coalition Building Between Public Health Nurses and Parish Nurses," *Journal of Nursing Administration* 23 (1993): 17-31.

3 Phyllis Solari-Twadell, Anne Djupe and Mary McDermott, eds., *Parish Nursing: the Developing Practice* (Park Ridge, Ill.: Parish Nurse Resource Center, 1990).

4 "Granger Westberg: Parish Nursing's Pioneer," *Journal of Christian Nursing* 6, no. 1 (Winter 1989): 26-29 **(in Chap. 10 of this publication)**; McDermott and Mullins, "Profile of a Young Movement": 29-30; Solari-Twadell, Djupe and McDermott, eds., *Parish Nursing*.

5 Janice Striepe and Judith King, "Basics for Beginning a Parish Nurse Program," *Journal of Christian Nursing* 10, no. 1 (Winter 1993): 12-15 **(in Chap. 11 of this publication)**.

6 King, Lakin and Striepe, "Coalition Building": 17-31; Sandra Miskelly, "A Parish Nursing Model: Applying the Community Health Nursing Process in a Church Community," *Journal of Community Health Nursing* 12, no. 1 (1995): 1-18.

7 Francesca Armmer and Patricia Humbles, "Parish Nursing: Extending Health Care to Urban African-Americans," *Nursing & Health Care: Perspectives on Community* 16, no. 2 (1995): 65-68.

8 Sandra Bergquist and Judith King, "Parish Nursing: a Conceptual Framework," *Journal of Holistic Nursing* 12 (1994): 155-69.

9 Mary McDermott and Joan Burke, "When the Population Is a Congregation: the Emerging Role of the Parish Nurse," *Journal of Community Health Nursing* 10, no. 3 (1993): 179-90.

9

Nursing Through the Lens of Faith
A Conceptual Model

Lynda Whitney Miller

Is God restoring nursing to its Christian roots?" the *Journal of Christian Nursing* editor asked in the winter 1996 issue. Sitting in my farmhouse, staring at the computer screen's image of yet another page of my unfinished dissertation, I closed my eyes. A memory made me smile and nod in answer: "Yes!" That memory was of wonderfully eager expressions on the faces of many nurses who, to my surprise, shared my interest in looking at nursing's theoretical models from a Christian point of view. During the twenty-two-year gap between completing my MSN and enrolling in PhD studies, I'd had few "close encounters of the nursing theory kind." Now, I'm engrossed in nursing theory.

In September 1992 I came back from a conference where I'd met nurses who were doing parish nursing. At the next meeting with my graduate program supervisor, I told her, "I've found the kind of nursing I feel I could devote myself to for the rest of my life."

My enthusiasm prompted her to suggest, "Then why not see if you can work it into your dissertation?"

In the following months I pondered possible research projects and various nursing conceptual models with their underlying worldviews. Figuring out the foundational philosophical beliefs was difficult because nursing theorists rarely state them. After reviewing the nursing theory literature in general, and Christian nursing and parish nursing in particular, I was disappointed. If the historical roots of Christianity and nursing were so intertwined, where were the conceptual models suitable for Christian nurses working in a distinctively Christian context?

True, some of Florence Nightingale's writings connect concepts of health with God's laws in nature. And Virginia Henderson's model includes worship in its list of fourteen basic human needs. But because I couldn't find a model explicitly developed from a clearly Christian worldview, my dissertation topic became "A Nursing Conceptual Model Grounded in Christian Faith." My goal was to provide Christian nurses with something which, although theoretical and abstract, had practical implications for parish nursing and other practice settings. The "Miller Model for Parish Nursing"[1] is the result of my conviction that conceptual models are important.

The Importance of Conceptual Models

Many nurses (including some of my friends and colleagues!), do not see nursing theory development as important to them personally. But then, before I started this project, neither did I. I remember with chagrin the time a school of nursing faculty member asked me, a new instructor, "Which nursing theorist's model do you use in *your* practice?"

I was doing casual work as a gerontological nurse in an extended care facility and was beginning an independent practice of health promotion workshops in the community. "Hmmm . . . Gee . . . Well, uhhhh . . . The self-care one—Orem's?" I stammered. I was embarrassed to realize how little awareness I had of my theoretical grounding and how much difficulty I had talking about it.

Before becoming an ABD (not an abdominal dressing but a grad student who has completed all-but-the-dissertation), I viewed nursing theorists as a select group of brilliant scholars, of interest only to academics expected to learn about or teach the various theoretical/conceptual models. Now I know that every nurse holds certain views or ways of seeing things which affect how that nurse practices nursing. So a nurse's conceptual model, which may be either more or less conscious, and more or less consistent, provides direction in the personal and professional attitudes, decisions and actions of daily nursing worklife.

Every nursing conceptual model presented in nursing literature describes its particular ways of viewing one or more of what could be called "the big four" components: a) person, b) health, c) nursing and d) environment. Seeing how nurse theorists have formally expressed their particular views through their published models can help other nurses express their own views informally.

Conceptual models are intentionally and, by definition, necessarily, highly abstract. From these broadly abstract models, nurses must derive more narrow and concrete nursing theories that may, in turn, be translated into more specific or practical terms, a process often called "operationalizing." Thus, parish nurses shouldn't expect to be able to apply my model directly. Application requires additional intermediary stages of developing more specific nursing theories. I hope that further thinking about the Miller Model by nurses, nurse educators and researchers will stimulate this process.

The Miller Model of Parish Nursing

The underlying worldview of the Miller Model of Parish Nursing is evangelical Christianity. Figure one shows "the big four" components of my model: 1) person/parishioner, 2) health, 3) nurse/parish nurse and 4) community/parish, plus, in the center of the window, the core integrating concept of the triune God: God (Father)/Christ (Son)/the Holy Spirit. The theological concept of the triune God, or trinity, is a Christian truth, affirmed across twenty centuries of church history, which unifies Christians amid cultural and denominational diversity. The centrality of this concept most clearly distinguishes my model from others. Figure one also shows the two major organizing concepts within each component.

When asked "Do you believe in God?" many will say yes. But, because individual perceptions of God may differ greatly, the parish nurse might then ask, "What God do you believe in?" or "How would you describe God from your perspective?"

In my model I've tried to describe the *personage* and the *purposes* of God as revealed in the Bible. The Bible says: 1) The triune God is a personal God, in intimate, loving relationship. God is also sovereign, good (righteous), just and merciful (gracious). 2) In the beginning, the triune God created everything good, intended for harmonious relationships. Since the Fall, restoration of relationships is made possible through Christ's life, death, resurrection and ultimate return. 3) The Christian gospel is *good news* because God did for humans what they could not do for themselves by providing a way through Christ to restore relationships (Heb 9:14-15, 22, 26; 1 Jn 4:10).

The **person** component in a nursing conceptual model is particularly important because a nurse's beliefs about human nature (one's own and others') affect how that nurse works with people. Also the nurse's viewpoints on human health, aging, illness, suffering, healing and death impact nursing care.

Current nursing models generally define *personhood* in terms of the individual as autonomous self. Most also reflect a secular humanist worldview in which the human self is central, with no existing external, transcendent, sacred "higher power." What distinguishes my model is not that it acknowledges a holistic body-mind-spirit view of person, for others do as well. And many models allow for spiritual care of persons by incorporating spirituality within their broad psychosocial or culturally sensitive approaches.

In my model the spiritual is central, and *personhood* is defined as a spiritual relationship with the triune God. The premise here

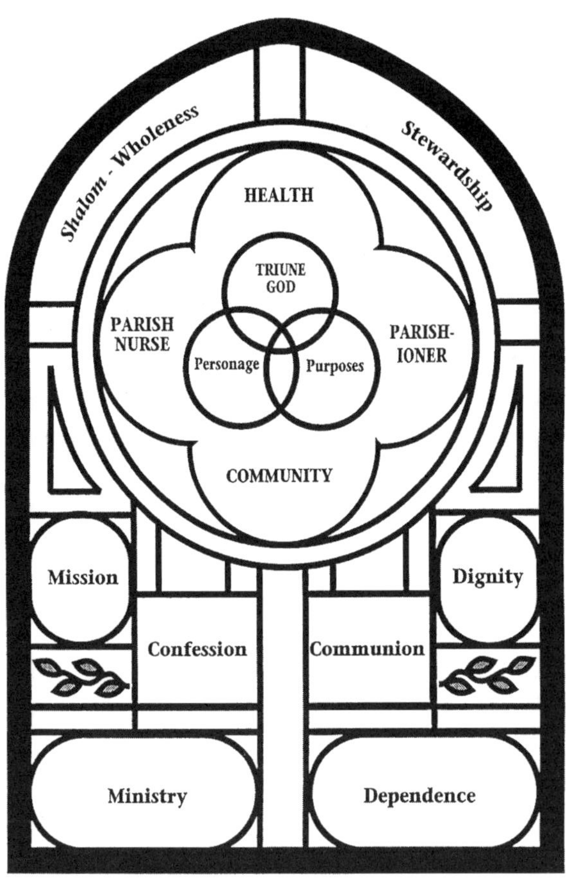

Figure 1: Components and major concepts of the model.

here is that the Christian gospel transforms people, providing them more than just a Christian system of thought or philosophical worldview. Two major concepts of my **person/parishioner** component are *dignity* and *dependence*. Human dignity includes such related concepts as personal worth, respect, inherent value and self-esteem. Dignity derives from 1) The special creation of humans "in the image of God" (Gen 1:27). Human reflection of that divine image has been distorted by the Fall, making everyone now a "a fallen image bearer."[2] 2) The unconditional love of the triune God toward all people (Jer 31:3) and the special covenant love relationship with those who accept the gospel of Christ (Jn 3:16; Rom 5:8).

The broad concept of *dependence* on the triune God as the ultimate Source and Sustainer of all life includes two more specific concepts: pardon and presence. Rather than acknowledge utter dependence on God, fallen image-bearers may assert self-sufficiency. However, when people repent (turn from going in the wrong direction to following God), God forgives them (Acts 10:43; Heb 10:16-23).

To acknowledge dependence on the triune God does not negate personal responsibility. In this model, people are viewed as responsible participants in promoting their own health. But, unlike other models, they are not expected to do so by their own power (physically, psychologically, socially or spiritually), but by drawing on the power of the triune God.

Although Christians are assured of God's love and pardon, the daily reality of living in a fallen world brings feelings of fear and powerlessness. All Christians (parish nurses and the persons they serve) experience the tension of living, both physically and spiritually, in the overlap of two contrasting worlds: the temporal, sin-afflicted present and the eternal past-present-future. Viewing the disorder and distress in this world through the eyes of faith in the sovereignty of God and his kingdom helps make some sense of it. Christians struggling with crises, illnesses or tragic life experiences can be encouraged and comforted by the active presence of the triune God, providing strength, peace and hope.

Figure two (page 66) suggests the complex and interrelated aspects of the person as an *inspirited* whole, and some health promoting resources.

I've defined the **health** component of the model in terms of biblical *shalom-wholeness* and *stewardship*, based on these key points about their inter-relatedness: 1) In the Old Testament the Hebrew word *shalom* has been translated as "wholeness" or "salvation." In the New Testament, the same Greek word meant "saved" in a theological context, and "made whole" or "healed" in a medical context. Our current English noun "health" and the verbs "to heal" and "to make whole" have also come from one Anglo-Saxon term. 2) "Sickness" or "disease" is a disruption of any dimension of wholeness, and "healing" is restoration of wholeness or fullness of human experience, not of the physical body only.

Within the **health** component, biblical *shalom-wholeness* and *stewardship* are defined separately, but the concepts overlap. "Stewardship" means being entrusted with something valuable and being accountable for managing wisely whatever one has received from God, including being disciplined in living a healthy lifestyle (1 Cor 4:1-2; 1 Tim 4:7-8; 1 Pet 4:10-11). Ideally, human stewardship reflects the triune God's compassionate concern for the well-being of all creation. And, again ideally, health as biblical *shalom-wholeness* is dwelling at peace and in harmony in all relationships: within oneself, with God, with other people and with the created, natural world.

Using the metaphor of Christ as a vine and believers as fruit-bearing branches (Jn 15:4-11), *shalom-wholeness* can be seen as arising from the vital relationship of the individual branches with the central vine. Thus, it is this model's view that personal *shalom-wholeness* is possible only through personal relationship with Christ. Ultimate well-being of the human community (full completion of God's *shalom*) will come only as part of the peace

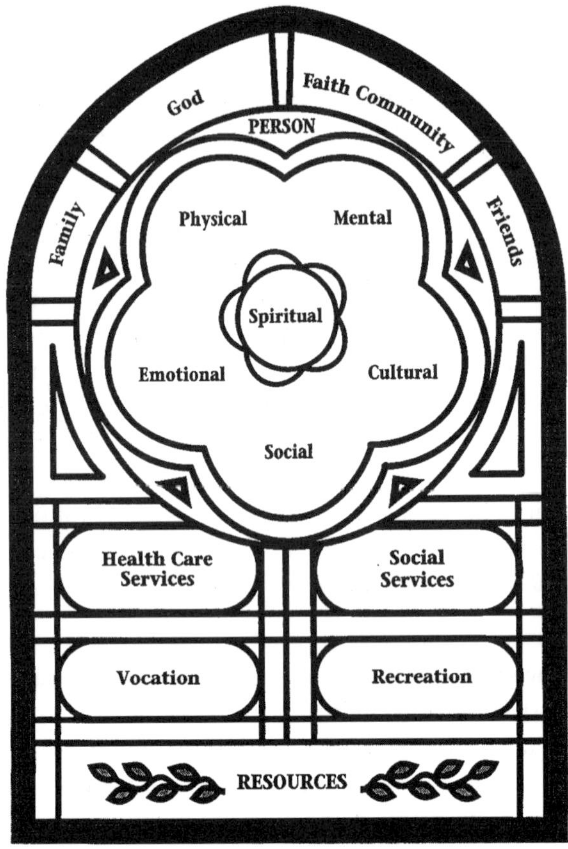

Figure 2: Aspects of the whole person (spiritual, physical, mental, emotional, social, cultural) and health promoting resources of the person.

and harmony of all creation after the return of Christ in the future "new heaven and new earth" (Rev 21:1-5).

The **nurse/parish nurse** component of the model reflects the fact that the Christian faith is both philosophical and practical. Thus, the major concept of *mission* includes the philosophical *why* and undergirding motivation of Christian nursing in general. The other major concept, *ministry*, covers the pragmatic *what* and *how* of parish nursing practice. Viewing parish nursing as a Christian calling is one expression of mission. A calling is calling is more than a personal sense of duty to do one's job or an awareness of human need. Ideally, the caring of the Christian nurse is a selfless serving that resembles that of Christ and is rendered to Christ.

Jesus modeled a radically different way of being with people than the accepted norm of society then and today. He related to each person with the respect shown between equals, the concerned interest between neighbors and the love between friends. It is this mutual service to one another that Christ directed his disciples, and us as Christian nurses today, to do (Mk 10:43-45; Lk 10:36-37; Jn 13:14-15; Phil 2:5-7).

Jesus' ministry involved preaching, teaching and healing. The parish nurse's ministry does too. Four additional primary concepts of the model, central to the nurse's various specific roles and functions, are love, gracious compassion, co-participation and spiritual care.

Finally, **community/parish** is a component of contexts. As shown in figure three (page 69), each context is viewed from the individual parish nurse's perspective. The parameters of the particular parish nurse's roles determine who and what that respective parish is. Each parish is unique.

The primary context is the local church congregation, including both people and church-related activities. A second context is the larger parish with which the local church is identified denominationally and/or ecumenically. *Parish* in this sense is generally defined in terms of geographical regions or organizational structures. At a higher level, a Christian context is the church worldwide. An additional factor is the immediate context of the sociocultural community, including cultural norms and public and private sector resources relevant to parish nursing.

The concept of *confession* in the model refers to two different activities identified with membership in a faith community. One is the profession of belief in certain doctrines, or a specific declaration of faith. The second is the admission of sin and seeking of forgiveness, which we've already discussed. It has been said that "Christian faith is intensely personal, but it is not private."[3] Personal beliefs are shared in common with Christians across continents and centuries, including the approximately 1.7 billion other members of the Christian church worldwide today. Great diversity is evident in what aspects of faith are emphasized and in how they are expressed, but unity of agreement on the core set of major tenets of Christian faith far outweighs doctrinal differences on more minor points.

The concept of *communion,* like "community," implies sharing in common and interrelatedness. Communion in this model is described in terms of the covenant relationship between the triune God and God's people, *koinonia* relationships among Christians and collaborative relationships between church members and the wider community. The New Testament's references to the Christian church, both general and local, as the "body of Christ" reflect the corporate nature of the covenant relationship with the triune God (Eph 5:29-30, 32; Col 1:24-29). Christians are bonded by their common faith in Christ into a family. The development of such close relationships implies spending significant time together, not only in worship, but also in work and play.

Health and healing are integral to the historic Christian church's *mission* and *ministry*; when local church congregations emulate Jesus' example and teachings, they are by definition communities of health and healing. Churches are concerned about both the health of their members and the health of the communities in which they are located. As stable and respected institutions in society, representing all social strata, they provide social as well as spiritual resources for individuals and families across all ages and life stages. Congregations promote health in philosophical ways by nurturing spiritual values and in practical ways by sponsoring health-related programs that can have an impact on the health of people and their environment.

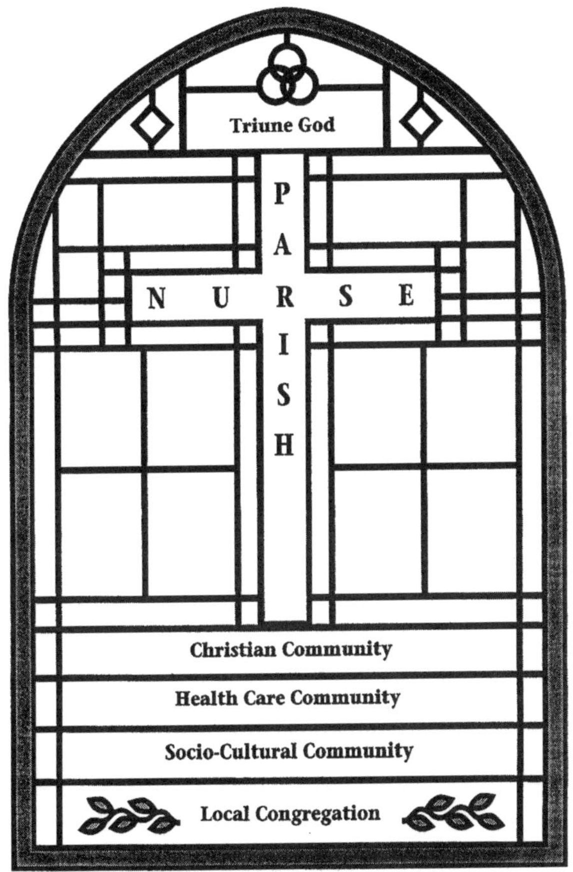

Figure 3: Contexts of the parish nurse role.

I've described it is, like parish nursing, a work-in-progress. I pray that you will join with me, the many parish nurses and others who want to participate in God's restoring of nursing to its Christian roots.

Originally published in JCN, Winter, 1997

NOTES

1 Lynda Whitney Miller, "A Nursing Conceptual Model Grounded in

NOTES

[1] Lynda Whitney Miller, "A Nursing Conceptual Model Grounded in Christian Faith" (PhD diss., University of Victoria, 1996).

[2] Lawrence J. Crabb, *Understanding People: Deep Longings for Relationship* (Grand Rapids, Mich.: Zondervan, 1987), p. 112.

[3] Peter C. Moore, *One Lord, One Faith: Getting Back to the Basics of Your Christian Faith in an Age of Confusion* (Nashville, Tenn.: Thomas Nelson, 1993), p. 8.

10

Parish Nursing's Pioneer
An Interview with Granger Westberg

Ramona Cass

Granger Westberg has done pioneering work in the area of religion and medicine. Trained as a pastor, he has taught at various seminaries and medical schools, including the University of Illinois College of Medicine and the University of Chicago. He is the author of The Parish Nurse. *A number of years ago he founded a series of clinics called Holistic Health Centers to treat physical ailments in the context of overall physical, spiritual and emotional health. Later he focused his energies on meeting whole-person needs through nurses who work in churches. That's what we talked to him about in this interview. Dr. Westberg died February 16, 1999.*

Why did you start the parish nurse program?

Nurses have special gifts that no one else has. I wanted those gifts to be used for the benefit of the church. And I saw that thousands of nurses are frustrated in their jobs because they aren't allowed to use their creativity in helping people.

Of the million-and-a-half nurses in America, only about a third are working. The others quit to raise families or because they were sick and tired of hospital systems that kept them from really spending time with people.

But parish nurses minister to both the physical *and* spiritual needs of people in a congregation. They exercise their people skills and caring personalities. Nurses command a special kind of respect from people, and they have an advantage over others when it comes to making it easy for people to open up about their problems.

What is the essence of the parish nurse concept?

It's really the culmination of my work in relating theology and health care. So let me explain how the idea came about.

In 1940 I pastored a church in Illinois. One day at a Lutheran pastors' conference in Chicago, several other young ministers and I sat with the seventy-year-old chaplain of Augustana Lutheran Hospital.

In the course of our conversation, this chaplain explained that he needed to be away from the hospital for a week. "Would one of you fellows like to take my place?" he said.

"I'd like to do that," I said. "I think it would be fun." That was the beginning of one of the greatest weeks of my life.

What was so memorable about the experience?

I was able to minister to patients effectively in a very short time. When people are lying horizontally in a hospital, they begin to think about the vertical dimension of life. They wonder about the meaning of life and start asking spiritual questions. But usually no one is around to help them deal with those difficult questions, so they don't get far with their thinking.

All during that life-changing week, I came in contact with people who needed help to think deeply and productively. I hope I helped them, as I injected biblical concepts into their thinking.

Just over three years later, as a result of contacts made that week, I became the chaplain at Augustana. That was 1944. I was thirty years old then, and people were just beginning to see the potential for changing lives through hospital ministry.

Over the years, ministering and teaching at Augustana and then the University of Chicago, I began to see that a person's physical well-being was tied to his or her emotional and spiritual health. Again and again as I talked to patients, I found that their illnesses seemed to originate in some personal struggle, often related to grief. (It was during that time that I wrote my book *Good Grief*.)

I felt that the key to preventive medicine lay in picking up people's early cries for help. Someone needed to be on the scene in the church to deal with people before they became seriously ill.

Is that how the wholistic health centers came about?

Yes. The first one began in response to the need for health care in a poor community. We opened a free clinic in a church, signed up two volunteer doctors and one volunteer nurse and used seminary students to do counseling. Subsequently we set up clinics in middle- and upper-income communities where people paid standard fees for the services. A nurse, doctor and pastor would treat these people's complaints holistically, recognizing that their problems stemmed from and affected not only the body, but also the mind and spirit.

But these clinics were expensive to start and operate. We had to pay the salaries of three or four professionals and the cost of renovating a building. And we had to subsidize the operations because we couldn't charge a high-enough fee to cover the expenses of treatment by three people instead of just one. However, a dozen of these clinics are still in operation across the country.

How did the parish nurse idea develop from this holistic approach to health?

I realized that the nurse was the key member of the professional team in these clinics. [So far all of them have been women.] She had the sensitivity—the peripheral vision, I call it—to see beyond the patient's problems and verbal statements. She could hear things that were left unsaid. And she was the best listener.

For example, when we would conduct initial interviews with patients, it was the nurse who really heard what was said. Then afterward she would give feedback to the doctor and the pastor: "Do you remember when Mrs. Olson was starting to tell you something, and you butted in and gave a little sermonette, Doctor [or Pastor]? She had something important to say, I think, and you stopped her."

Nurses seem to have one foot in the sciences and one in the humanities, one foot in the spiritual world and one in the physical one. The nurses I've had the privilege to work with have been very perceptive; they have great insight into the human condition.

What do you think makes them that way?

Many of the nurses I work with have a deep spiritual desire to help people. They don't view the hospital as a warehouse for sick bodies. They see people as sacred in God's eyes. Consequently, they look at the whole person, not just the ailment.

When many doctors enter a patient's room, too often they view the patient with a sort of tunnel vision. They see the physical problem and nothing else. If the patient has something wrong with his or her arm, doctors will go right to the arm, take care of it and leave. Maybe they spend only a few minutes with that person. In many cases they say almost nothing to the patient beyond asking about physical symptoms.

But nurses entering the same room will see and hear a great deal more than some doctors. Nurses may comment on pictures or get well cards, or talk with the family members who've come to visit—all at the same time that they are caring for the patient's physical needs.

One day, while lamenting the expense of running a holistic health center, a friend said, "You were saying such wonderful things about nurses. Instead of opening a clinic, what if we just put a nurse on the church staff? Would that work?"

We tried it, and it worked. Then I approached the president of Lutheran General Hospital in Park Ridge, Illinois, an old friend of mine. We discussed the concept of the parish nurse as a practitioner in preventive health care. He was as excited about it as I was. So we decided to test the idea in six Chicago-area churches—four Protestant and two Catholic.

How did that work?

The six churches each chose a nurse. We gave them a list of applicants, and the congregations also had women who were interested in the positions.

Lutheran General agreed to sponsor the program by paying 75 percent of the half-time salary for each nurse the first year. The second year the hospital paid 50 percent, and 25 percent the third year. Thus each year Lutheran General paid less, and the churches paid an increasing percentage of their nurse's salary. By the fourth year, each church was paying the nurse's full salary.

Each year, as the hospital reduced its contribution for the original six nurses, we added two more churches to the program with the extra money. Now we have twelve churches.

What kind of preparation do these nurses receive?

We set up a low-key continuing education program at Lutheran General. Once a week the nurses meet for half a day with me, the chaplains, a nurse from the hospital teaching program and a doctor in family medicine. These people provide support and guidance for the nurses.

When we get together, the nurses share stories about their ministry. Sometimes they role-play things that have happened during the week. They exchange ideas about ways to handle problems, and they have fellowship together and with the hospital chaplains.

What sort of things do the nurses do at the churches?

First, they are health educators. They hold seminars, workshops and discussion groups. Over potluck suppers and in Sunday-school classes, they teach people to take care of themselves. The nurses don't do all the teaching. Often they bring in doctors or other professional people to talk about health care as it relates to the spiritual life. Most of these professionals have never before been invited to lecture in a church, where people ask questions about faith.

The parish nurses frequently take parishioners' blood pressures. That way they easily get to know people. Often someone will come up to a nurse after church and say, "Could I talk to you later about some personal things?" Thus nurses have a special point-of-entry to develop relationships.

That brings me to another role of parish nurses: They are health counselors.

The elderly usually come to the nurses first. They bring questions about medications or physical problems that they don't want to call the doctor about. Discussions about physical problems will frequently open the door to talking over other issues.

Then parents will come to the nurses because a teenager has a problem with drugs or alcohol. The nurses can help them personally and set up special seminars for other parents dealing with difficult teens.

Later, maybe a year later, men begin to approach the nurses. That's where nurses really have an advantage over other people. Men are taught not to ask for help. But it's okay to ask a health care professional about a physical problem. So, men make appointments to talk to the nurses about physical problems and end up discussing other things.

It happens over and over again. A man comes in to see a nurse about his back pain. When they're finished, the nurse expects him to leave, but he doesn't. Instead he stays and stays and talks and talks—about all kinds of things in his life. He finally leaves saying, "I've never felt free to talk to my doctor or even my minister. It's easy to talk with you."

Why do you think men are so willing to talk to nurses?

Part of it relates to what I already said about health care professionals. People hold them in high esteem. The public knows that nurses have seen it all—the seamy side of life, suffering in hospitals, people stripped of all pretense. So people feel freer to tell nurses things that they wouldn't tell someone else.

Also, nurses are usually women, and men can talk more easily to women. Studies show that men don't usually talk to other men about personal matters. They talk about football or cars or basketball, but not personal things.

In parish nurses men find women who are scientifically trained, have seen the harsh side of life and are good listeners. The nurses are also kind, compassionate and knowledgeable. That's a combination men can relate to. Like women, men hold nurses in high esteem.

Most nurses don't feel that they are held in high esteem. If people really respect nurses so much, why don't they feel it?

I think that nurses feel unappreciated because most doctors don't express gratitude for the work they do. Some doctors look down on nurses. So nurses pick up that attitude and believe the public also fails to appreciate them. But I do not believe that's an accurate perception.

Just listen to people when they're talking about problems. You'll hear someone say, "Well, I talked to Mary Smith about that, and she's a nurse. She told me it probably wasn't serious." What nurses say carries great weight because people respect their knowledge. That's one big reason why we're using only nurses in this program.

I've had social workers and others come to me and say, "I could do that kind of work." Maybe. But they wouldn't have the special background that nurses have. Social workers might be as sensitive, and they might be good listeners. But they don't have the scientific expertise that nurses do, so they wouldn't command the same respect.

Nurses can attend church coffee hours, and by the end they'll have identified five people they want to visit that week to discuss something in more depth. Their peripheral vision has been at work picking up early cries for help.

We know that a third of all illnesses would not have gotten as bad as they did if someone had intervened in the early stages. People experiencing stress or grief might be able to avoid eventual physical problems if someone were there to help them early on. Nurses can do that. In addition, parish nurses train volunteers who then assist them, visiting people and providing for the personal and health needs of the congregation. The nurses also act as liaisons with other community services, making referrals, getting people involved in support groups, and relating to the staff of local hospitals and nursing homes.

Funding parish nurses must be very expensive. Are other hospitals willing to pay salaries for nurses to work in churches the way Lutheran General has done?

Admittedly, hospitals are cutting back these days. Yet some are committed to preventive health care, especially the religious hospitals like Catholic, Lutheran, Presbyterian, Methodist and Mennonite institutions. Sponsoring parish nurses is one way of doing preventive health care along with pastoral care. Lutheran General Hospital's program is funded by the pastoral care department.

We already have a hundred churches participating in parish nurse programs around the country, especially in Illinois, Iowa, Nebraska and California. About seventy nurses work several hours each week as volunteers. That has turned out better than I'd expected. In some cases churches started paying the volunteers when they discovered how valuable their work was.

What plans do you have for the future?

I'd like to have a thousand churches with parish nurse programs. We now have a Parish Nurse Resource Center at Lutheran General Hospital.[1] I'd like to have a full-time director to run that. And I'd like to see a special program for training parish nurses—either a six-week session at Lutheran General, or a staff member who would travel and train nurses on site.

Then I'd like to organize a parish nurse association to provide a newsletter and to set up local support groups for parish nurses. If I only had $35,000!

Originally published in JCN, Winter, 1989

NOTES

1 Lutheran General eventually became part of Advocate Health Care, which withdrew its support from the International Parish Nurse Resource Center (IPNRC) on Jan. 1, 2002. The IPNRC is now maintained by Deaconess Parish Nurse Ministries, 475 E. Lockwood Ave., St. Louis, MO 63119; phone: 314-918-2559; e-mail: arethemeyer@eden.edu.

Part Three:

What Does a Parish Nurse Do?

11

Basics for Beginning a Parish Nurse Program

Janice M. Striepe & Jean M. King

H.L. Mencken said, "For every complex problem or issue, there is a simple solution. However, it's usually wrong!" We would paraphrase, "For every question, there is a simple answer, but it is not always correct." What should you consider if you are asking the question "Should I be a parish nurse?" Admittedly, the answer is not simple, but by hearing stories of other nurses' experiences, you will see the positive aspects of the complex and diverse methods involved in starting a parish nurse service.

Jan's Story: Congregation-Based Model

When I became interested in parish nursing in 1984, I talked with my pastor about being a parish nurse at Trinity Lutheran Church (350 members), and I spent many hours over four months laying the groundwork. There were no parish nurses in our rural area, and I wanted to ensure that our members, as well as the health and social work professionals, understood the role.

I wrote a proposal to our church council, outlining the role and my responsibilities for a five-hour-per-week parish nurse position. Since our church was unstable financially, I asked only for office space (I do not recommend this approach!). The council accepted the proposal, and I began communicating with community health nurses, social workers, physicians and other key professionals in our area, informing them about the parish nurse role, asking if they had any questions and listening to their comments. All reacted positively.

In our church I talked to various committees and groups, as well as asking members to complete an interest survey before a worship service. All expressed high interest in health education programs. I reviewed tools for record keeping and adapted them for my new parish nurse role. I wrote a parish nurse brochure, started a pamphlet library, wrote church newsletter articles, and read holistic health books and Bible studies about health and healing. My pastor and I planned together. I wanted to focus on two priority projects. We decided on a holistic health series for the adult Sunday school, followed by a series on grief.

We also felt that a special program, Individuals of Wholistic Awareness (IOWA), would be beneficial. Members who enrolled in IOWA would attend the health series, meet with me to write personal holistic health goals, and confer with me regularly for support and guidance. IOWA was a good kick-off activity for the new ministry. Other nurses choose to promote their parish nursing with special events such as a health fair or an intergenerational program. One church with ample funds purchased copies of the book *Seeking Your Healthy Balance* by Donald and Nancy Loving Tubesing (Whole Person Associates, Duluth, Minnesota, 1991) and gave a copy to each family on the Sunday of the parish nurse's installation service.

During my first year as a parish nurse, the Social Ministry Committee agreed to expand its goals to include health, creating the Social and Health Ministry Committee. Later the congregation approved my request for Trinity to enroll in Iowa Lutheran Hospital's Minister of Health Program. I would attend their classes and be salaried for twenty hours per week (half being paid by the hospital) for one year. Although my education, teaching and community health experience were a good basis for the parish nursing role, I wanted to learn more, especially about Clinical Pastoral Education. Every year since has brought new programs and opportunities for learning.

Jean's Story: DCE Model

I first became involved with parish nursing in 1986 when Jan asked if I would be interested in assisting her in the development of educational programs for the Northwest Aging Association's (NAA) Parish Nurse Project funded by the W. K. Kellogg Foundation. I have continued to be associated with parish nursing in the areas of education, evaluation, research and resource development. Although I do not serve as a parish nurse in my 2,400-member Catholic church, I have been involved in faith sharing and other activities.

Various nurses have been interested in serving as a parish nurse in this church since 1986, but for various reasons, the time was not right for them. Pastoral leadership has changed, and there is increasing emphasis on lay ministry and community building within the congregation. Parish staff has expanded to include pastoral ministers, a youth director and a director of Christian education (DCE).

Often church staffing includes a DCE. When a job description is developed for this position, it could be advantageous to select a registered nurse. The combined role of the DCE and parish nursing has evolved successfully in some churches in northwest Iowa. The nursing activities, which include caring, community building, nurturing, and healing and wholeness, would complement religious education and theology. A major advantage of this model is that it provides the opportunity to incorporate the entire congregation in the activities and interventions formerly reserved for children and youth.

Sally's Story: Co-Parish Nurse Model

When a member of my church and I read an article about parish nursing, we were convinced that this was needed in our 200-member church. During our planning phase, we decided that we would share the position of parish nurse. We wrote a proposal describing which activities each of us would be doing and a schedule of who would be there for the parish nurse office hours. We have developed a special friendship as we support each other in a shared parish nurse role.

Evelyn's Story: Team Model

I have a busy family and work schedule. But I've always been a teacher and a youth group leader, plus being involved in other church activities. When my pastor talked to me about parish nursing, I was excited, although also frightened and a bit overwhelmed. Over the weeks and months, a great team model evolved in our 600-member church. Because of the support and interest of other nurses and health professionals, I decided to be the parish health coordinator and to decrease my other church responsibilities. I work four to six hours each week planning, communicating and coordinating, plus visiting my foster grandparents.

Since the parish nurse job is broad, we decided to divide and conquer the role. Many nurses agreed to have a foster-grandparents relationship with one to five frail elderly members. Other nurses agreed to do one of the following activities: 1) send get-well, sympathy and thinking-of-you cards to persons on the three-, six-, nine- and twelve-month anniversaries of the death of a loved one, 2) monthly blood pressure checks, 3) hospital and nursing home visits. An OB-GYN nurse volunteered to visit church families who had a newborn.

Some of the health professionals wanted to be involved only intermittently. I contact them for members who have short-term needs and for group presentations.

I utilize the youth group and women's circles for assisting members. For example, a family needed respite assistance because the pregnant mother was on bedrest and could not care adequately for their three-year old. Since they had limited financial resources, they were thankful that I could arrange volunteers for three hours each morning to care for the child and do light housekeeping.

Team members record their activities on a form, and I compile them on a master report form that is given to the council. For our church, this model has worked well, and I'm thankful that we have been able to serve our congregation and community.

Community Models

There are two types of community models in our network. In Marcus, Iowa, population 1,200, each of the five churches has a parish nurse. Obvious advantages are support, sharing expertise, referring clients to each other, offering programs together and increased cooperation among the churches.

An important aspect of this model has been the development of community outreach programs. With all the churches cooperating on a project, they are able to help more people and identify community health priorities. When the need for a long-term care facility was recognized, the nurses and pastors were key people in the community's success in obtaining a certificate of need to build a nursing home.

The other community model involved two or more churches cooperating to hire one parish nurse. In one town, the two local denominational leaders simply met and agreed on the action. In another city, the ministerial association decided that each of its member churches would contribute money to hire a nurse.

The Non-Parish Nurse Model

Most nurses will never become official parish nurses. However, may nurses have told us what they do in their congregations. Even though they are not parish nurses, they are catalysts for holistic health and for enhancing caring in their churches.

Hearing about parish nurse activities and interventions has inspired nurses to be more intentional about using their nursing skills for fellow Christians in their local churches. For example, nurses have become Stephen Ministers, have led occasional health programs or have facilitated an exercise class.

Mary's Story: Barriers

When I learned about parish nursing at a conference, I began exploring my options. I encountered several barriers during the planning stage. At the conference, the presenter stated that usually a parish nurse is an RN with at least two years of nursing experience, but there is no nationally recognized certificate and no standards of practice nor educational requirements for parish nurses. Since I am an LPN with a degree in health education, I was unsure if I could call myself a parish nurse. Because of my work experience, I felt comfortable in the parish nurse role but did not want to be reported to the Board of Nursing for practicing outside the role of an LPN.

The problem was solved when an RN in our church agreed to supervise, guide and support me. Other LPNs have told me that they do not call themselves parish nurses; they are care coordinators in their churches.

My pastor was supportive, but he was so busy that he wanted me to present the idea to the church leaders. My first presentation met with lukewarm response, and they had many questions. I suggested several actions: 1) I would give each of them articles about parish nursing to read; 2) at the next meeting, I would show the video *The Connecting Link*; and 3) at the following monthly meeting, I would have a parish nurse talk to them, using the speaker system on our phone so they could all hear her. It would have been better to have a parish nurse in person, but none were nearby.

After laying this groundwork, I had enthusiastic support, which enabled me to continue with my planning. Two other barriers that needed to be addressed were accessible training and concern about liability. Using money from the Memorial Fund for tuition and expense, my church sent me to the three-day conference in Chicago sponsored by the Parish Nurse Resource Center. My pastor and I alleviated members' fears about being sued by assuring them that I carried professional liability insurance and that the church would purchase a policy specifically designed for parish nurse service. Pastor also gently but firmly suggested, "Yes, we could get sued; however, that should not be a reason to deny this ministry." Since I focus on wellness activities and do not do physically invasive nursing procedures, the probability of being sued is low.

During the planning process, I learned how important it is to patiently listen and inform. Because I did not push members to make a quick decision, they felt ownership of the new service, as well as being supportive.

Issues: Funding

In our experience, we have found funding to be the major issue. It would be ideal if all parish nurses would be salaried. But the reality is that not all churches can accommodate this type of expenditure. Once the congregation commits to establishing a parish nurse program, options can be explored.

The pastor or nurse could contact the chaplaincy department of the local hospital for financial support or for sponsoring educational classes. Other institutions that have supported parish nurse networks are denomination-based nursing homes and colleges. Fraternal insurance companies and individual denominational district, regional or state offices have been funding sources. One example: the Health and Welfare

Committee of the Iowa Conference of the United Methodist Church has budgeted money for parish nurses.

To spur interest in a collaborative, community-based network, the pastor or nurses may ask a hospital or college to sponsor a workshop on parish nursing. Community partnerships have often led to cooperative funding for a network.

Other options for funding include special church offerings and church fundraisers, which have the advantage of involving members. Some networks have received grants from private foundations. Your local library will have a book that lists and describes all charitable foundations.

More than one nurse has written a proposal stating that he or she would be a volunteer parish nurse for one year, with the stipulation that the church provide funding after that, if the program is to be continued.

Sometimes none of these ideas are successful or feasible. Being a volunteer has its advantages. Many nurses who have been both a volunteer and salaried have said, "When I was a volunteer, any activity was greatly appreciated, but when I became paid staff, the expectations for activities and interventions were much higher." Church members often make unrealistic demands on their paid staff. Whether the nurse is salaried or not, a health ministry will need funds for resources and expense reimbursement. Any ministry requires some funding to be effective.

Being a Parish Nurse Pioneer

In the book *The Parish Nurse* (Augsburg, Minneapolis, 1990) Granger Westberg gives steps to start a parish nurse program. He writes that you need to: 1) learn all you can, 2) inform and talk with the pastor and key leaders, 3) form a health committee, 4) try to establish a link with a hospital, 5) select and orient the nurse, and 6) begin the program.

In addition, we think that it is important to use the nursing process to determine the most appropriate model. Doing a reflective and detailed assessment of yourself, the pastor and leaders, the congregation and community, will help you decide your planning, implementation and evaluation strategies, as well as deciding which model of parish nursing will work best in your church.

Throughout the process, remember the power of prayer. Request that prayer be offered during the worship service, as well as utilizing your personal prayer time and other previously existing avenues for prayer in the church.

There are no easy, simple steps to starting a parish nurse service. Parish nurses repeatedly say that the developmental process proved to be necessary and beneficial. They enjoy being pioneers. Parish nurses exemplify the saying "Don't go where the path leads; go where there is no path and leave a trail."

Originally published in JCN, Winter, 1993

12

What Does a Parish Nurse Do?

Rita P. Wilson

The revolutionary changes taking place in the health care system are having monumental effects on institutions, personnel and recipients of health care services. These changes include cost consciousness among health care providers and recipients, which prompts concerns about quality of health care.

People are exhibiting an increased sense of responsibility for promoting and maintaining good health and preventing illness, plus a growing concern about access to quality, affordable health care. With the proliferation of options available and the fragmentation in the health care delivery system, many are feeling overwhelmed and confused about how to meet health care needs. The health care system changes have increased the need for specially trained professionals who can help individuals and families move through the system to address their needs. The professional nurse has always been central to that system and, in a time of change, has the potential to be key in enabling clients to access the systems and utilize available resources.

One setting for providing health care to specific populations, which has come into focus in recent years, is the church. The goal is to provide holistic health care to a church community. The parish nurse provides client services not generally offered. Traditional health care models concentrate on physical and psychological influences to the body but tend to neglect the spiritual realm. The parish nurse cares for clients as a whole: body, mind and spirit.

This model is based on the following concepts: 1) The person is a whole being made up of body, mind and spirit; these facets interact with each other to maintain optimum health. 2) Health is an evolving process, continually working to maintain balance. 3) Holistic health focuses on prevention. 4) Holistic health includes self-care; clients are responsible for their own health. The health care provider and the client work together as a team to maintain optimum health. The central mission of the parish nurse and the church is restoration. The nurse and the church actively engage with the living Creator in reclaiming and healing the whole of creation.[1]

The Christian Medical Commission of the World Council of Churches states: "Our vision is that all will understand, live out and celebrate the healing restoration of the integrity of God's creation through a process in which the human spirit and the Holy Spirit work together to heal relationships to God, self, family, community and creation as a whole."[2]

The parish nurse functions as a community health nurse who also becomes God's representative of love, caring and healing on earth. The church becomes the nurse's community, in which wellness is promoted by holistically addressing members' physical, emotional and spiritual needs. The parish nurse model illustrated on page 94 depicts the nurse as the focal point who connects individuals and families with resources to provide care to a congregation over life's continuum: physical birth, new life—being born again in Christ, suffering—the pains and sorrows of life, surrender—to God's grace and mercy, physical death and resurrection—everlasting life in glory with Christ.

Health can be described as maintaining an optimal level of wellness and wholeness. Parish nursing is based on the biblical concept of wholeness expressed by the words *shalom* in the Old Testament and *peace* in the New Testament, meaning well-being, health, happiness and harmony. The words imply the healing of all fractures between man and God, man and man, man and nature, with nature, and among man, nature and God.[3] The biblical "holistic health" is harmony between a person and God, the source of healing and well-being.

With this focus in mind, the Parish Nursing Continuity of Care Model emphasizes harmony in mind, body and spirit. Through this model, the professional Continuity of Care Nurse exhibits caring along the congregation's health continuum. The

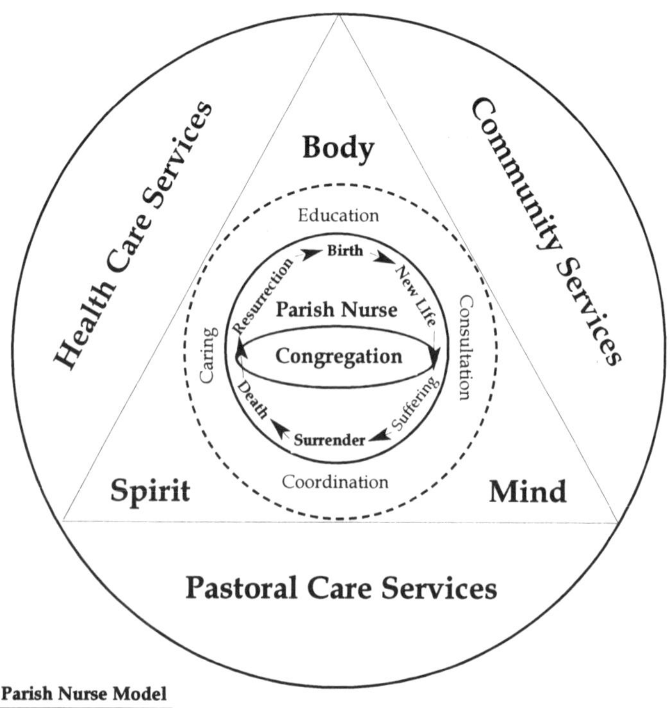

The Parish Nurse Model

nurse is the pivotal point connecting the needs of the congregation and resources over life's continuum *(Parish Nurse Model, page 94)*.

Who Is the Parish Nurse?

The parish nurse is a blend of caring, compassion and healing, providing consultation, education and caring that is enveloped in the healing spirit of the Lord. The nurse functions in the three levels of care: primary, secondary and tertiary, for the church through birth, new life, suffering, surrender, death and resurrection.

The parish nurse's role may include 1) **education**: providing illness information and offering classes on a wide range of health and wellness subjects [4] and teaching responsible self-care regarding emotional, physical and spiritual health.[5] 2) **consultation**: advising individuals and groups about physical, emotional, social and spiritual concerns[6] and making home, hospital and long-term care visits as needed. 3) **leader of individuals and groups**: organizing and supervising volunteers from the congregation to assist with parish nurse activities, and developing and leading self-help groups. 4) **coordination**: making referrals to physicians and community support services,[7] assuring member access to and use of appropriate community health care resources and serving as advocate for the congregation to other health care providers.

The role of the nurse has always been caring for the sick and needy in the community. Caring is central to the parish nurse practice because it conveys to clients a sense of importance as individuals and connectedness to life.[8] Parish nurses actualize the faith community as a caring body by mobilizing and working with church committees, pastors and parish volunteers to assist members in need.[9]

The parish nurse's role may vary from congregation to congregation, being defined by the expertise and strengths of the parish nurse, the support of the pastoral staff and the needs of the faith community. Parish nurses are key to the local congregation's health care, as they become involved in all phases of the members' lives at all age levels, periods of development and at times of joy and sorrow.

Who Is the Congregation?

The core of the model is the individuals and families within the congregation: clients of a variety of backgrounds, ages and socioeconomic levels. The elderly may call on the parish nurse for information about medications, diet, hospitalization, living arrangements, grief and loss. Middle-aged adults may have questions about parenting, marital relationships and health problems. The parish nurse can address concerns about substance abuse and adolescent sexuality, as well as teach sessions on healthy eating, stress management and domestic violence. The parish nurse may do home postpartum visits with instruction on care of newborns, or visit homebound clients to offer reassurance and spiritual support, as well as home assessment, dressing changes and health teaching.

Clients of the parish nurse's practice may be outside the faith community, coming through referrals from church members or other health care professionals. Health care programs offered to the broader community can serve as an outreach ministry. Health fairs, blood pressure screening and meals for the homeless may be provided in collaboration with other community agencies.

What Is the Parish Nurse Practice?

The goal of parish nursing is to promote holistic health and well-being by enhancing the sense of harmony with mind, body and spirit within the faith community. This is depicted in the Parish Nurse Model (page 94) by the points of the triangle. Any of the three may require intervention by the nurse in the form of educating, consulting, coordinating and caring. A parish nurse must be a generalist in nursing practice to function from a broad knowledge base. Utilizing the nursing process and advanced nursing knowledge, the parish nurse can help clients access community resources, pastoral care and health care services.

The Body: Physical Health and Wellness

Parish nursing activities support physical health and wellness and include health promotion and prevention activities, restorative care, self-care and referrals. Classes on wellness, first aid, parenting, violence prevention and developing exercise programs are examples of prevention activities. Health programs need to include the spiritual aspect traditionally overlooked in other health care settings.

Specific prevention activities may include personal health risk appraisals, health pamphlet libraries and well-elderly clinics provided in conjunction with community health agencies.[10] Blood pressure, hearing and vision screening may be offered to the church family, as well as to the outside community and can serve as an opportunity for the nurse to share the gospel.

Restorative activities may include home visits, home meals programs and referral to community resources such as transport services or meals-on-wheels for those discharged from the hospital. The nurse also acts as an advocate for those wishing to remain independent at home by assessing their needs and striving to meet those needs. Clients who are hospitalized sometimes report that they are able to return home earlier than otherwise would be possible because of parish nurses' advocacy and referral to appropriate community resources.[11]

The parish nurse promotes self-care by educating clients on risk factors for heart disease, cancer or stroke. Clients are encouraged to become responsible for personal lifestyle changes that can reduce their risk factors. These activities increase the clients' understanding of disease processes and empower them to take responsibility for their own health. As awareness of healthier lifestyles increases, more individuals come to parish nurses for information and consultation.[12]

The Mind: Emotional Health and Wellness

Emotional health and wellness activities may include educational programs that address wellness and incorporate the spiritual aspect. Potential activities include 1) social support, especially with the elderly dealing with loss, grief and feelings of isolation and loneliness, including encouraging, touching and praying, and 2) organization of support groups and classes on stress, violence, conflict resolution and time management. The parish nurse may refer clients to support groups within the community such as *Mended Hearts*, an Alzheimer's support group or an organization for eating disorders.

The parish nurse can help the client to regain a sense of self-worth and dignity. Clients report feeling less lonely, having their fears of grief and loss alleviated and feelings of helplessness decreased because of visits with the parish nurse.[13] God's caring is demonstrated through the parish nurse's practice. The act of caring helps others to grow to their fullest potential.

The Spirit: Spiritual Health and Wellness

Because the spiritual component of nursing practice is often missing in traditional health care, addressing spiritual health is a vital component of the parish nurse practice. The parish nurse needs to be sensitive to the spiritual realm and guided in practice by the leading of the Holy Spirit. To develop a holistic plan of care, the spiritual aspect must be interwoven with the physical and the emotional aspects.

The parish nurse's activities may include providing spiritual assessment, offering to pray, reading Scripture and discussing specific religious issues with the client. Parish nurses can assist pastors in identifying the spiritual needs of the congregation as they explore clients' relationships with God. Jointly examining purpose and direction in life is a part of a holistic evaluation.[14]

As a spiritual caregiver, the parish nurse may make formal presentations to the church. Further nursing activities to support spiritual health and wellness include values clarification, compassion and provision of faith and hope.[15] Individuals may renew, regain or reaffirm their relationship with God and others as a result of the spiritual care given by the parish nurse.[16]

The strength of parish nursing lies in personal spiritual discipline and continued practice in the ministry. The parish nurse can be a valuable asset to the congregation in meeting physical needs and assisting the clergy with the congregation's spiritual direction. Granger Westberg described the spiritual aspects and goals of the parish nurse as: 1) maximizing the healing heritage in the Christian tradition in the sacraments, fellowship, support groups and educational groups, thereby experiencing grace that is healing and 2) ministering with and beyond the realm of medical technology and its systems to assist the church to fulfill its role in the healing of all aspects of creation.[17]

Services: Health Care, Community and Pastoral Care

Collaborative practice with other health care providers, community agencies and the church's pastoral staff is necessary for the parish nurse to accomplish the goal of holistic health care for clients. In the Parish Nurse Model (page 94), these major service areas are depicted immediately within the outer circle of the model. Parish community members may access the health care system and be referred to other health care providers. They may also be connected with community services for the purpose of seeking funding for outreach projects, obtaining educational resources and participating in support groups. Pastoral services are essential to assist in meeting clients' spiritual needs. The nurse's role complements the pastoral services of the church to offer in-depth spiritual care and enhance clients' personal spiritual growth.

Collaborative relationships are the foundation of parish nursing practice. These relationships are a positive force for effectively meeting the goals of clients and the nurse, developing cooperation within the community and improving comprehensive health care.

Thus we see that parish nursing provides holistic care and practical service, as well as integrating the concepts of health and healing into the faith community over the continuum of life. It is based on a continuity-of-care model that provides for the delivery of holistic care. Parish nursing optimizes the physical and emotional aspects of individuals, families and communities by incorporating the spiritual aspect.

The concepts of congregation, nurse, health (body, mind, spirit) and the nursing process create a framework for organizing the concept of parish nursing. This framework can provide a format for implementation of a parish nurse program and for parish nurse practice. Further conceptual development and validation of the components within the framework may be provided by future nursing research.

Originally published in JCN, Winter, 1997

NOTES

1 L. James Wylie, "The Mission of Health and the Congregation," in *Parish Nursing: The Developing Practice*, Phyllis Solari-Twadell, Anne Djupe and Mary McDermott, eds. (Park Ridge, Ill.: National Parish Nurse Resource Center, 1990), pp. 11-26.

2 John Gilnett, "To Your Health," *Response* 14, no. 2 (1991): 4-5.

3 Jan Striepe, *Nurses in Churches: A Manual for Developing Parish Nurse Services and Networks*, (Spencer, IA: Northwest Aging Assoc., 1989).

4 Phyllis Solari-Twadell and Granger Westberg, "Body, Mind and Soul: The Parish Nurse Offers Physical, Emotional and Spiritual Care," *Health Progress* 72, no. 7 (1991): 24-28.

[5] Jean King, Jean Larkin and Jan Striepe, "Coalition Building Between Public Health Nurses and Parish Nurses," *Journal of Nursing Administration* 23, no. 2 (1993): 27-31.

[6] Granger Westberg, "Parishes, Nurses and Health Care," *Lutheran Partners*, (Nov./Dec. 1988): 26-29.

[7] Solari-Twadell and Westberg, "Body, Mind and Soul": 24-28.

[8] Jan Striepe and Jean King, "Is Caring the Essence of Spirituality?" in *Proceedings from the Fifth Annual Granger Westberg Symposium: Faith, Spirituality and Caring, the Essence of Parish Nursing* (Park Ridge, Ill.: Nat. Parish Nurse Res. Ctr., 1991).

[9] Jan Striepe, "The Developing Practice of the Parish Nurse: A Rural Experience," in *Parish Nursing: The Developing Practice*, P. Solari-Twadell, A. Djupe & M. McDermott, eds. (Park Ridge, Ill.: Nat. Parish Nurse Res. Ctr., 1990), pp. 129-46.

[10] Anne Djupe and Robert Lloyd, *Looking Back: The Parish Nurse Experience* (Park Ridge, Ill.: Nat. Parish Nurse Res. Ctr., 1992).

[11] Jan Striepe, Jean King and Linda Scott, "Nurses in the Church: Profiles of Caring," *Journal of Christian Nursing* 10, no. 1 (1993): 8-11 **(in Chap. 14 of this publication)**.

[12] Djupe and Lloyd, *Looking Back*, p. 29.

[13] Linda Scott and Jack Sumner, "How Do Parish Nurses Help People? A Research Perspective," *Journal of Christian Nursing* 10, no. 1 (1993): 16-19 **(in Chap. 13 of this publication)**.

[14] Richard Fehring and Marilyn Frenn, "Holistic Nursing Care: A Church and University Join Forces," *Journal of Christian Nursing* 4, no. 4 (1987): 25-29 **(in Chap. 19 of this publication)**.

[15] JoAnn Boss and Jennifer Corbett, "The Developing Practice of the Parish Nurse: An Inner-City Experience," in *Parish Nursing: The Developing Practice*, P. Solari-Twadell, A. Djupe and M. McDermott, eds. (Park Ridge, Ill.: Nat. Parish Nurse Res. Ctr., 1990), pp. 77-103.

[16] Marcia Schnorr, "Spirituality Caregiving: A Key Component of Parish Nursing, " in *Parish Nursing: The Developing Practice*, P. Solari-Twadell, A. Djupe and M. McDermott, eds. (Park Ridge, Ill.: Nat. Parish Nurse Res. Ctr. (1990), pp. 201-20.

[17] Granger Westberg, "A Historical Perpective: Holistic Health and the Parish Nurse, " in *Parish Nursing: The Developing Practice*, P. Solari-Twadell, A. Djupe and M. McDermott, eds. (Park Ridge, Ill.: Nat. Parish Nurse Res. Ctr., 1990), pp. 29-37

13

How Do Parish Nurses Help People?
A Research Perspective

Linda Scott with Jack Sumner

When I first read about parish nurses, I thought, *This is the direction that I want to go – to search, to know more about them and what they do.* As I continued to read and talk to individual nurses involved in parish nursing, it became an interest area full of pleasant surprises. I soon developed a deep respect for parish nurses. But it wasn't until I began doctoral studies that I understood the significance and importance of the work of these practitioners.

Psychology and applied medicine have done extensive interdisciplinary research on the relationship of the mind and body, with various theories and treatments of psychosomatic illness gaining and waning in popularity.

As I studied parish nursing, I appreciated the emphasis on a vital connection between mind and body—the spirit. My reading on parish nurses and my doctoral study brought me to the same point. Parish nurses are able to connect and draw things together in meaningful ways for their clients. They bring their knowledge, experience and skills to meet the client's needs.

Parish nurses effectively couple diverse and disparate components in a way not usually observed in nursing practice. The outcome of that coupling is generally positive, particularly when it deals with the merging of holistic needs, and the end result is holistic nursing care.

The Project Begins

My expanded exploration of parish nursing began with a partnership consisting of Jan Striepe and Jean King from the Northwest Aging Association's (NAA) Parish Nurse Project; my dissertation adviser, Dr. Jack Sumner; and a group of University of Iowa RN/BSN students. Assistance for the doctoral study came from the NAA Kellogg-funded project in Spencer, Iowa. The parish nurses from each of the sixty-three parish nurse services in western Iowa were selected as the population.

Little research had been done on outcomes related to parish nursing, so I felt further investigation and follow-up could build on the results of this study. I was interested in finding out the clients' perception of the care they had received and wanted to know what they would say about holistic health care and the helpfulness of the nurses. I had to find out what parish nurses did for clients and see how that related to the perceptions of the clients about the care received.

Because of significant geographical distance between the clients, the parish nurse project site and my location, a qualitative approach of working with observations and descriptions, rather than depending on large numbers, seemed to be the best method.

Using an interview guide to record responses, eight students from a nursing research class through the University of Iowa assisted me in talking on the telephone to forty-seven clients. The 155 *yes* or *no* questions, plus five that were open-ended, could be covered in a twenty-minute interview. Clients were also queried about their backgrounds.

In assessing the holistic care received from the parish nurse, questions included: 1) fifty-four about physical care, 2) forty-seven about emotional care and 3) thirty-four about spiritual care. The content of the questions in each of the three categories included: 1) the client's concern or problem that led to seeking out the parish nurse, 2) the client's perception of what the nurse did and 3) his or her thoughts about the results of the interventions.

Results of the Project

An expected finding was the high percentage of elderly females, sixty-one and older, who used the parish nurse service—almost three-fourths of the total number of clients interviewed. Most of the parish nurse services in western Iowa are located in predominately rural areas, which have a high percentage of elderly residents.

Because parish nurses are health promoters and educators, another expected finding was that clients frequently utilized the parish nurse service for this reason. Three of the four top priority concerns for clients were desires to know or learn something about their health or disease. All the clients who came to the parish nurse because of a concern about their illness or condition said they gained the sought-for understanding. Most (92%) said that because of their visit with the parish nurse, they had healthier lifestyles.

Anxiety, learning to deal with emotions and loss of health or bodily functions were the three most frequently reported emotional problems or concerns that clients discussed with the parish nurse. All who brought emotional concerns believed that the parish nurse satisfactorily provided supportive measures by listening, consoling and encouraging. All the clients felt that they learned how to problem-solve and felt less lonely. Most were comforted (95%), had their fears of grief and loss alleviated (90%) and feelings of helplessness decreased (88%) because of their visits with the parish nurse.

The spiritual aspect of parish nursing proved to be more obscure, less clearly identified by the clients and less frequently reported than either the physical or the emotional aspect. Only about half the clients said they discussed spiritual topics with the parish nurse, such as healing, God's presence and hope (51%). Nurses initiated discussion on faith and belief in God, according to half of the clients. The most commonly reported nursing interventions were the acknowledgment of their beliefs (73%) and encouragement of their faith in God (67%). Improved feelings of well-being was the most frequently reported spiritual consequence (85%) of the client's visit with the parish nurse.

Parish nursing was well received by the clients, and their responses about the service were overwhelmingly positive. "A caring, compassionate person, enjoyable to visit with," characterized the client's view of the parish nurse. Clients could call the parish nurse at any time, and that availability was important to them. They appreciated having a parish nurse accompany them to appointments with the physician and help them to access the complex health care system.

Clients readily identified physical reasons to go to the parish nurse, but they were less apt to see the nurse for emotional or spiritual concerns. However, once their physical problems were cared for, the parish nurse helped them to identify related emotional and spiritual needs. Because everyone has a spiritual dimension to help overcome physical problems, holistic care touches a broad range of human experiences.

The Spiritual Dimension

Spiritual care is what makes the holistic approach of parish nursing different from any other nursing specialty. Parish nurses need to develop this aspect more fully. The findings indicate that nurses do provide spiritual care, but it tends to be more passive in nature, such as accepting the clients' beliefs. More active spiritual care interventions would include reading Scripture, praying with or for clients, and laying-on hands. These could be a part of almost every nurse-client interaction and would provide a unique added dimension to the more usual health-promotion type of nursing care. These interventions have the potential of making a significant difference in people's lives.

For those who use the parish nurse service, it seemed that their positive response was related to their view of parish nursing as an extension of the church. Since the church was already a vital part of their lives, they naturally accepted the parish nurse and the service provided.

Outcomes Personalized

All I had learned about parish nursing outcomes became intensely personal. During the time I conducted this study, I was dealing with my own experience of holistic care. My mother was diagnosed with an inoperable brain tumor, and my family chose to care for her at home. Although the physical care consumed a great deal of time, we tried to balance it with emotional and spiritual care. Daily Bible reading, prayer and singing together softened her attitude toward her illness and anticipated death.

Our pastor taught me about the spiritual dimension of care—how and what to pray, appropriate Scripture and the laying-on of hands—and I was amazed at the difference it made, not only for Mother, but for our whole family. I decided that the spiritual care my mother and our family received was definitely within the realm of the parish nurse and should be emphasized in their preparation. This experience personalized my understanding of parish nursing and helped me to realize the consequences of holistic care within the total health-care system.

Originally published in JCN, Winter, 1993

14

Nurses in the Church
Profiles of Caring

Janice M. Striepe, Jean M. King & Linda Scott

I'm so thankful that Pastor and I could be a caring team for Mary. It's been six months since her teenage son died in a car accident, and we were able to help her understand the physical, emotional and spiritual aspects of grief." These comments are typical of those made during the parish nurse share-time meetings.

As parish nurse coordinators, we are renewed by hearing the comments and reliving the joys and sorrows in the experiences of the parish nurses participating in the education classes and share-time meetings. Their caring activities bolster our pride in nursing and our belief that Christian nurses are healers. Their stories validate the parish nurse role as an important emerging specialty.

Profile of a Developing Practice

Parish nurses are registered nurses who initiate a health care ministry in a church setting to assist congregational members in their physical, emotional and spiritual wellbeing. The ministry is rooted in Scripture, specifically Jesus' command to "proclaim the kingdom of God and to heal" (Lk 9:2). We use the acronym HEALTH to describe their role.

Parish Nurse Role

H	Health Counselor
E	Educator of Wholistic Health
A	Advocate/Resource Person
L	Liaison to Community Services
T	Teacher of Volunteers/Support Groups
H	Healer--Body, Mind and Spirit

When we began coordinating parish nurses in 1986, we underestimated the interest of both pastors and nurses. The Northwest Aging Association (NAA) in Spencer, Iowa, began with twelve parish nurses. As of 1989, the W. K. Kellogg Foundation provided funding to expand the network. By 1991 we were assisting sixty-three parish nurse services in western Iowa. In 1992 the network had grown to ninety parish nurse services.

NAA's network is a community-based project relying on the collaborative efforts of religious, health, social and educational institutions and professionals. In the network we provide a stipend, resources and educational classes. The churches provide office space and furniture. Some churches provide expense reimbursement and/or salary. The collaboration has contributed greatly to the success of the program.

But the most important factor in the project's success is the nurses. When beginning her parish nursing practice, one nurse said, "I may not know exactly where I'm going, but I'm sure not lost!" Nurses have functioned as informal community or parish nurses for years, answering health questions from family, friends and church members. We found that informal parish nursing was particularly common in smaller churches in rural communities.

However, there is a definite transition from that informal parish nursing role to an organized health ministry in the churches. For instance, it is important for the nurse to work with a standing church committee such as Social Ministry, Christian Education or Missions to establish a health committee. One nurse said, "There are so many needs—the elderly, single parents, health promotion screening and information, many stressed people. I don't know where to start and how to prioritize." Educational classes prepare and guide the nurse, as well as assisting her in setting priorities.

Since the parish nurse role is multifaceted, we encourage the nurses to develop their services based on their personal strengths and interests, as well as a congregational needs assessment. Knowing that nurses often neglect their own needs, we remind them that *being* (taking time for prayer, meditation, Scripture reading and their own holistic growth and balance) is as important, sometimes more important, as *doing*. On the monthly activity report form, we have a section to rate their holistic health for the month and write comments.

Profiles of the Nurses and Churches

We were amazed at the diversity of data (ages, backgrounds) of the sixty-three nurses. Their ages range from twenty-nine to sixty-six, with the majority (54) between thirty-one and sixty. All the nurses are female, and all but one are or have been married (four were widowed; six divorced). One nurse is an African-American, and the rest are Caucasian. Most of them are employed part- or full-time in more than eleven areas of nursing, usually in a hospital. Thirty-three are diploma- or associate degree-prepared nurses, and thirty have a BSN or higher degree. Thirty-five live in towns with less than 5,000 people; fourteen live in towns of 5,001 to 15,000; and fourteen live in a town with more than 15,000 residents. Nearly all (61) serve in their own churches.

Most said they became parish nurses so they could combine their faith with nursing practice. One nurse commented,

"Parish nursing gives me the opportunity to work with the whole person, including physical, emotional and spiritual health, and to focus on teaching wellness, wholeness and optimum health." The majority indicated that the most satisfying aspects of parish nursing are their personal growth and the meaningful, deep relationships with clients.

The sixty-three churches in NAA's network show great variety. Eleven denominations are represented, with the Lutheran, Methodist and Catholic churches in the majority. This is understandable since these denominations are the most numerous in the area and have been leaders in promoting parish nursing. The congregational membership ranges from fifty to 2,800. More than half (37) have less than 500 members.

The majority of the churches (53) reflect western Iowa's demographics in that more than twenty percent are elderly members, and over half of those fifty-three churches have more than forty-one percent elderly members. Although our area is predominately Caucasian, there is a growing number of Laotians, Hispanics and other minorities locating in western Iowa.

Activities and Intervention

We have compiled activity data about the sixty-three parish nurse services for two years, from January 1990 to December 1991. The bar graphs provide a summary of the client contacts (figure two), reasons for the contacts (figure three), and the ages of the clients (figure four). The elderly concern category refers to a "sandwich generation" person who has a concern about an elderly friend or relative. In addition to the client contacts at church, home or by phone, the nurses have done more than:

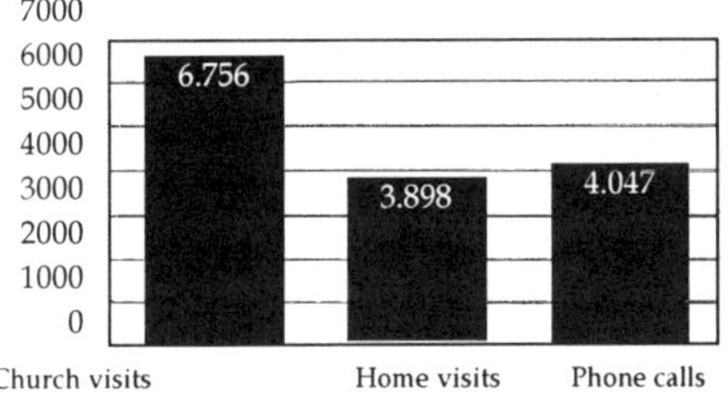

figure 2. Two years 01/01/91—12/31/92 = 14,701

- 600 health promotion programs
- 2,000 referrals to health/social professionals
- 500 support group meetings
- 3,800 greeting cards
- 850 articles
- 8,400 blood pressures (7,700 normal and 750 referred)
- 1,900 coordination meetings
- 2,000 hospital and nursing home visits

We found it interesting that programs about stress, nutrition, exercise and holistic health were the most common. Grief and loss classes were also held frequently.

The nurses have organized special events, such as health fairs (29) and training sessions for lay visitors (113). They have provided or arranged for transportation for 323 clients. Their interventions have assisted 125 elderly to remain at home, instead of moving to a health care facility.

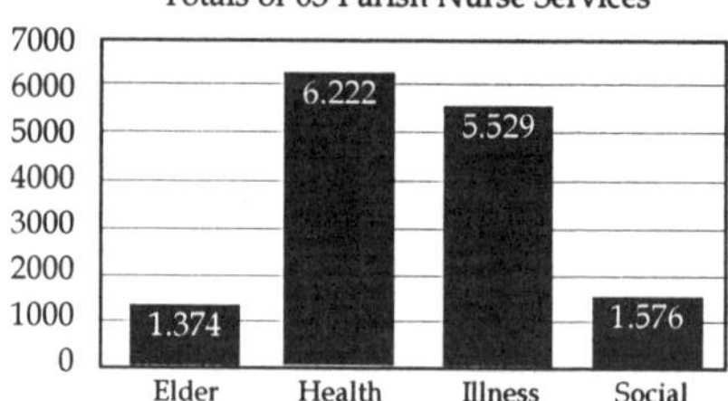

figure 3. Total client contacts = 14,701

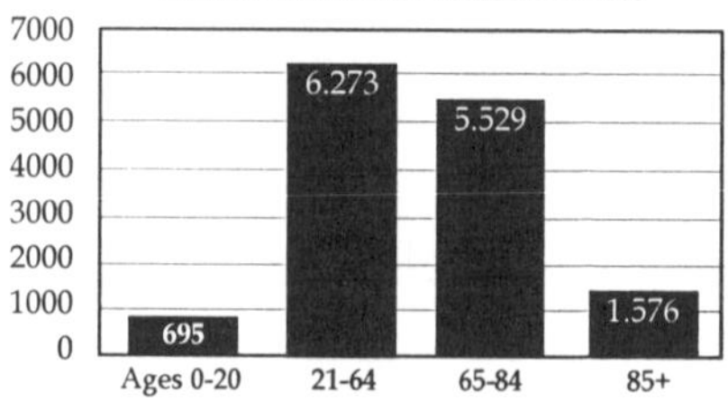

figure 4. Total client contacts = 14,701

Parish nurses have supported church members during times of change and loss. They have helped elderly clients to move from their homes to nursing or retirement centers. This assistance is especially appreciated by those who have no family in the community. The nurses help people to understand grief by offering classes, providing pamphlets and by organizing support groups. Many of the elderly cannot travel miles to a larger town that has a grief support group, but they can easily meet after the worship service for support and fellowship with others in the congregation who have lost a loved one.

Why are these numbers important? They demonstrate that people do respond to the parish nurse service. But it is the nurses' experiences of increasing holistic care that are the most important. Their stories of caring and making a difference in the quality of life are the essence of parish nursing.

One nurse wrote, "Sam came to me in tears. He said, 'Matilda is better after her stroke, but now the doctor says she has to go to a nursing home. Can you help me? I want to take care of her at home on the farm.' I assured Sam I would do my best. I called the physician, and though he was not willing to refer Matilda to the Metropolitan Stroke Rehabilitation Center, he did not object to my exploring other options. After I made several phone calls, she was admitted to a nearby center.

"When she was ready to be discharged, I worked with the center's nurses and the social worker on the home-care plan for Matilda and Sam. Our local physical therapist and community-health nurse taught Sam transfer techniques and special procedures, since Matilda, a diabetic, was in a wheelchair and had a Foley catheter. Community-health nurses and homemakers provided personal care three times a week. I arranged for church members to visit regularly.

"One month later, her mind, body and spirit literally glowed from pride in her own persistence and the strength she received from God. I thanked God as I watched her give her own insulin as Sam looked on proudly. His eyes filled with tears when he said, 'They say she will be walking with a cane before long!'"

Positive comments from pastors also validate the parish nurse concept. They appreciate the nurses' caring efforts. One pastor said, "Not only has our congregation become more of a caring community, but our nurse supports me and reminds me to take care of myself. She has helped improve the quality of my family life by encouraging me to take time for my wife and children."

In 1984, Lutheran General Hospital in Park Ridge, Illinois, began the first network in the U.S. with about twelve parish nurses. By 1992 there were over fifty networks and 1,500 known parish nurses. Although the Midwest has the most of any area in the country, parish nurses are serving in rural, urban, suburban and inner-city settings throughout the country.

Granger Westberg, the father of the parish nurse concept, stated in the Winter 1989 *Journal of Christian Nursing*, "Nurses have special gifts that no one else has." We heartily concur. We know he is both thankful and amazed at how the number of parish nurses and networks has grown.

Originally published in JCN, Winter, 1993

15

What's a Parish Nurse to Do?

Congregational Expectations

Lisa J. Mayhugh & Karen H. Martens

Although parish nursing is often promoted as a new field of nursing, it is actually a revival of an old model. Throughout nursing history, we see religious orders and church congregations providing care for the sick. Faith communities have been involved in the delivery of health care for more than 2,000 years. Parish nursing began as early deaconesses provided holistic care to those most in need. Christian mission has always included healing activities for the widowed, the children, the sick, the lonely and the poorest of the poor.

However, contemporary parish nursing started in 1984 with Granger Westberg, a Lutheran minister, who is credited with the idea of a congregation-based health ministry.[1] He believed that the church could play a bigger role in health by using church-based nurses to promote health and healing.

Sixty-five percent of the U.S. population belongs to a faith community.[2] People frequently turn to their ministers for help and see spirituality as a way of coping with stressful events. Parish nursing is an updated form of caring for the body, mind and soul of a person. Parish nurses help individuals define their states of harmony or disharmony and teach them how to care for themselves and others. I Peter 4:10 says, "Like good stewards of the manifold grace of God, serve one another with whatever gift each of you has received." Parish nurses exhibit the grace of God through caring for people in a faith community.

Westberg's pilot parish nurse program began seventeen years ago, and today approximately 6,000 parish nurses practice within the structure of a faith community. In recent years, some hospitals have begun to provide education and support for parish nurses. One example, the *Body and Soul Parish Nurse Program of Community Hospital* in Springfield, Ohio, was begun in 1997 and currently supports twenty churches and about fifty parish nurses.

As coordinator, I (Lisa) provide consultation to churches interested in initiating a parish nurse program. In addition, we provide new parish nurse programs with a variety of equipment: blood pressure cuffs of various sizes, first aid kit, stethoscope, drug book, CPR mask, printed educational materials and materials for record keeping. I make presentations to church boards as requested and provide monthly educational meetings for the nurses. We offer a yearly parish nurse seminar in cooperation with another local hospital.

With the growing interest in the specialty, parish nurses are beginning to build a solid base of research data. With both a personal and professional interest in parish nursing, I wanted to know more about outcomes of parish nursing. So this became the focus of my master's thesis. The purpose of the study was to identify the scope and effectiveness of one parish nurse program as described by one church's congregation, pastor and parish nurses. A model for parish nursing as developed by Rita

Wilson provided a framework for organizing survey questions and analyzing data.[3]

The church studied has about 200 attending the Sunday morning worship service. The church has had a parish nurse program with three active volunteer parish nurses for five years. All persons twenty-one or older were invited to complete a survey on one Sunday morning. The survey asked which services the parish nurse should provide, what services currently provided at the church the participant had used and which were helpful. Participants were also asked to agree or disagree with statements about parish nursing and program offerings. Additional written comments were also invited.

Sixty-seven church members plus six parish nurses and the pastor completed the survey. Over half (54%) of the church members who responded were sixty-one or older and a majority (79%) were female and married (73%). All parish nurses were female and married. Four were between forty-one and sixty, and two were under forty-one. Three nurses have a diploma in nursing, two have an associate degree in nursing and one has a BSN. The nurses were experienced, having practiced an average of twenty-two years and participated in parish nursing an average of four years. The pastor was male and fifty-five.

Preferred Services

Dividing the parish nurse roles into the four described by Wilson (education, consultation about problems, visiting [caring] and coordination—see table, page 118), participants were asked which services they preferred. Overall, people thought parish nurse services should focus on helping people to stay well and to manage physical or emotional disease. While over half thought the parish nurse should offer education about spiritual health, less than a fourth thought the parish nurse should consult about spiritual problems.

Services most preferred (80%) were educational with content about staying well and health screening. Several persons said that they preferred group classes as opposed to one-to-one education, noting the value of group interaction. Over half of those responding also wanted the parish nurses to visit people who were terminally ill, after hospitalization and at a nursing home. A *chi* square analysis determined that persons who were younger than sixty preferred that parish nurses visit after births and during and after hospitalization significantly more than persons greater than sixty ($p = < .05$). Also, those younger than sixty wanted education about emotional health and parenting more than did those over age sixty ($p < .05$).

Faith Community Preferences for Parish Nurse Services

Service	Congregation Women/Men	Parish Nurses	Pastor	Total #/%
Education About:				
Disease	22/9	5	1	37/50
Staying Well	44/8	6	1	59/80
Spiritual Health	31/4	6	1	42/57
Emotional Health	34/6	6	1	47/64
Violence	10/2	3	1	16/22
Health Screening	41/11	6	1	59/80
Parenting	16/4	3	1	24/33
Consultation About Problems:				
Physical	36/9	5	1	51/69
Emotional	30/8	2	1	41/55
Social	16/5	3	1	25/34
Spiritual	9/5	3	1	18/24
Visiting:				
After Births	22/5	6	1	34/46
After Hospitalization	29/9	6	1	45/61
Terminally Ill	38/7	6	1	52/70
At Hospital	14/2	4	1	21/28
At Nursing Home	27/4	6	1	38/51
Coordination:				
Train Volunteers	28/7	4	1	40/54
Develop/Lead Groups	24/5	3	1	33/45
Referrals	23/8	5	1	37/50

Table 1

Of all the programs offered by the parish nurse, blood pressure screening is the only one offered more than once. Blood pressure screening has been the one most attended (58% of those responding to the question). Attendance at other programs included: health fair (42%), a stress seminar (36%) and a class about fat-free meals (28%). Few attended a Bible school program (12%), glaucoma screening (8%) or an ethics seminar (6%).

Satisfaction with Parish Nurse Program

Only fifty-one persons (76% of the sample) responded to questions designed to evaluate the program. Of those, some participants did not answer all the questions. However, responses indicate that, overall, participants were satisfied with the parish nurse program. Two-thirds of the participants believed that the parish nurse program was a necessary part of the church. The program emphasizes educational offerings and provides other services to the church members. Fifty-one percent of the participants said that their parish nurse program has given them a sense that someone cares about them. Twenty-one percent noted that the parish nurse program helped them connect with pastoral care.

That the program is less involved in the area of emotional and spiritual care for its members seems to fit with the desires of the faith community. The subjects in this study were interested in education about spiritual health, but few wanted parish nurses to provide consultation for spiritual problems. Perhaps they associate such services with the pastor rather than with the nurses. Nurses often provide spiritual care, but it tends to be more passive in nature, such as accepting clients' beliefs.[4]

Janet Kuhn reported that when parish nurses were asked to describe how they incorporate spirituality into their role, they said they did such things as: praying with clients when it seemed right; taking Communion to clients; promoting wellness of body, mind and soul; showing compassion and caring for all; and discussing spiritual concerns during illness.[5]

The parish nurses believed that the program provided helpful information and was educational but was not highly visible at the church. Because the program is made up of volunteers, one nurse felt that it is adequate. Other nurses indicated that nurses could be more active as a committee and provide more services to the church. It is important to note that the pastor's responses to the survey, as well as his support of the program and allowing this survey to be conducted, indicate support of parish nursing. Such support is critical to the success of any parish nurse program.

Implications for Parish Nurse Programs

In traditional health care, the component of spirituality is most often missing, and that is why some believe that parish nurses must address spiritual health in their practice.[6] Parish nurses cannot be comfortable dealing with spiritual concerns unless they address their own values and belief systems and what gives their life meaning and purpose.[7] Paul states in Philemon verse 6, "I pray that the sharing of your faith may become effective when you perceive all the good that we may do for Christ."

If a faith community wants parish nurses to help them deal with their health in relation to spirituality, nurses must be adequately prepared. However, a parish nurse does not replace the pastor. Rather, the parish nurse helps people to see how health is related to spiritual health and assists the pastor in identifying the spiritual needs of the faith community, thus providing holistic care. Parish nurses are spiritual nurturers.[8] Such nurturing contributes to improved life satisfaction and quality of life, improved health, reduced functional disability and lower levels of depression.[9]

While this descriptive study examined only one parish nurse program, it was unique in that it sought responses from parishioners, pastor and parish nurses. This faith community has the greatest interest in services that help them stay well and identify and deal with physical health problems. This study reflects the importance of educating a congregation about potential services that a parish nurse program can offer, then assessing which services it needs.

All faith communities do not have the same needs. Because many parish nurse programs are staffed by volunteers, it is necessary to maximize those valuable resources by developing a program that truly meets the needs of the faith community.

Originally published in JCN, Summer, 2001

NOTES

[1] Lawrence E. Holst, "The Parish Nurse," *Chronicle of Pastoral Care* 7, no. 1 (Spring/Summer 1987): 13-17.

[2] Rosene M. Dunkle, "Parish Nurses Help Patients—Body and Soul," *RN* 59, no. 5 (May 1996): 55-57.

[3] Rita P. Wilson, "What Does a Parish Nurse Do?" *Journal of Christian Nursing* 14, no. 1 (Winter 1997): 13-16 **(in Chap. 12 of this publication).**

[4] Linda Scott with Jack Sumner, "How Do Parish Nurses Help People? A Research Perspective," *Journal of Christian Nursing* 10, no. 1 (Winter 1993): 18-20 **(in Chap. 13 of this publication).**

[5] Janet K. Kuhn, "A Profile of Parish Nurses," *Journal of Christian Nursing* 14, no. 1 (Winter 1997): 26-28. **(in Chap. 8 of this publication).**

[6] Wilson, "What Does a Parish Nurse Do?" **(in Chap. 12 of this publication).**

[7] Linda Miles, "Getting Started: Parish Nursing in a Rural Community," *Journal of Christian Nursing* 14, no. 1 (Winter 1997): 22-25 **(in Chap. 18 of this publication).**

[8] Beth Abbott, "Parish Nursing," *Home Healthcare Nurse* 16, no. 4 (April 1998): 265-67.

[9] Miles, "Getting Started" **(in Chap. 18 of this publication).**

Part Four

Models of Ministry

16

Mercy Model
Church-Based Health Care in the Inner City

Maria T. Boario

The Mercy Hospital Parish Nurse Program began in January 1991 as a mission-oriented, values-based community outreach program with seven part-time nurses serving ten congregations in the inner city of Pittsburgh, Pennsylvania. The first year of operation seemed truly miraculous, with the results clearly exceeding our original expectations.

The Mercy Hospital of Pittsburgh, a 524-bed inner-city tertiary hospital, provides an integrated health care system with a longstanding commitment to serving the needs of the poor. The teaching of the Roman Catholic church and the hospital's sponsors, the Sisters of Mercy, undergird its philosophy and practice.

Sister Joanne Marie Andiorio, RSM, DrPH, president of the Mercy Hospital of Pittsburgh and Pittsburgh Mercy Health System, learned of the parish nurse program at a Catholic Health Association conference and recognized the true healing ministry of this church/health care partnership. The vice president of mission services, Lawrence A. Plutko, consulted with the National Parish Nurse Resource Center® in Park Ridge, Illinois, and soon began dialogue with seven clusters of churches, all of which were located in medically underserved areas of Pittsburgh.

Hired as manager of the program in June 1990, I began my second week of orientation by visiting and talking with several parish nurses and program managers in the Chicago area. This orientation, arranged by the hospital in cooperation with the National Parish Nurse Resource Center,® provided valuable insights into the role of the parish nurse.

When I returned to Pittsburgh, I wanted to develop a parish nurse program that reflected the uniqueness of Mercy Hospital: its longstanding commitment to the poor, its integration of mission and values throughout the health care system and its visionary leadership in undertaking this creative outreach program. Above all, I wanted a program that would give glory to God, so I committed it to him. Ephesians 3:20 (LB) became my prayer: "Now glory be to God who by his mighty power at work within us is able to do far more than we would ever dare to ask or even dream of—infinitely beyond our highest prayers, desires, thoughts or hopes."

Next, I conducted needs assessments of each parish expressing an interest in the program. As I walked through the neighborhoods with the pastors, I became aware of the uniqueness of each congregation, as well as the social commitment that each pastor had for his neighborhood.

For various reasons, several churches declined to participate. Some pastors felt reluctant to start a new program because of the financial instability of their parishes; others wanted to take a wait-and-see approach; another did not see the need for a parish nurse.

After careful evaluation, ten congregations were finally selected—seven Roman Catholic, two Lutheran and one United Church of Christ—with memberships ranging from seventy-five to 3,000. Because of their geographic proximity and smaller membership, six churches would be served by three nurses. The four largest churches would each have their own parish nurse.

Parish Nurses Selected

Selecting the parish nurses became my next challenge. In undertaking a project of this size, I believed the key to our success would be in matching the right nurse with the right church. As I prayed that God would send a team of nurses for this endeavor, the truth of Romans 10:11-12 struck me: "The scripture says, 'No one who believes in him will be put to shame.' For there is no distinction between Jew and Greek; the same Lord is Lord of all and is generous to all who call on him."

In response to advertising in three Pittsburgh newspapers, as well as church bulletins, forty nurses applied. Surprisingly, no applicants came from the selected churches. No minorities applied either, although recruitment strategies targeted these two populations. The manager of the Pastoral Care Department and I interviewed twenty applicants and narrowed the field to fourteen finalists. The churches and their respective health committees then interviewed at least two nurses, and we mutually agreed upon the parish nurse for each church.

The hospital held a joyful and symbolic *missioning* service for the seven parish nurses. Sister Joanne Marie anointed each of the nurse's hands with oil, and the Reverend Abigail Rian Evans gave the keynote address, "Called by God." We felt a special bonding to our sisters in the Spirit, the Sisters of Mercy. One hundred and forty-four years after seven Sisters of Mercy founded The Mercy Hospital of Pittsburgh, seven parish nurses followed in their footsteps and tradition to provide holistic care to the inner city.

The orientation for these parish nurses was what my colleague Jennifer Corbett, OSF, at the Columbus Cabrini Parish Nurse Program, calls the plunge method. After three days of intensive in-service training, they went into the community to take the plunge. Weekly staff meetings provided peer support, collaboration/resource sharing and spiritual formation, besides the sharing of successes and frustrations. Our prayer list quickly grew to include clients, friends and families, those in authority over us, as well as ourselves.

The weekly staff meetings became a continuation of orientation and training as representatives from community agencies and Mercy Hospital came to discuss their programs and seek ways to collaborate and link resources. These resources and the expertise of skilled hospital professionals greatly enhance an institution-based parish nurse program. Nurse clinicians, physical and occupational therapists, and pharmacists, to name a few, graciously volunteer their time and talents to assist the parish nurses with community health presentations and health fairs.

The Nitty-Gritty of the Program

Being integrated into a health care system means that the parish nurses may receive merit pay increases based on performance goals that are written each year. While this process continues to be refined, we have, at times, struggled to preserve the primary purpose of the program—a healing ministry—while maintaining program accountability and overall hospital/corporate goals.

Program accountability means having a system for documentation of records, monthly reports, policies and procedures, as well as a quality assurance plan in accordance with JCAHO standards. Because we are accountable to our clients, to those in authority, and ultimately accountable to God, we see these mechanisms as positive developments in achieving program excellence.

Funding for the program comes from Mercy Hospital, from corporations, foundations, private contributors and from the churches served. We realized that the congregations chosen for our program would not be able to pay the salary of a part-time nurse; however, we felt it was important to develop a sense of ownership and partnership with the churches.

For the first year of operation, the churches contributed office space, telephones and secretarial support. They paid mileage for the home, hospital and nursing home visits made by the parish nurses. During that year, we hoped to demonstrate that a parish nurse, with all her nursing skills and spirituality, would greatly enhance and complement the congregation's ministry team. Now into the second year, the churches see the benefits and blessings of having a parish nurse and contribute financially to support the program.

Of the seven parish nurses hired, two are master's-prepared, two have BSNs and three are diploma graduates. Their special gifts and talents and spiritual maturity have been an inspiration to me and to the faith communities they serve. One of the parish nurses, a Presbyterian serving a Catholic parish, assisted in *the blessing of throats* on the Feast of St. Blaise one month after she began as a parish nurse. While the nurses give selflessly to their congregations, they are also learning to say no without feeling guilty. Setting limits is vital in preventing burnout.

The administration at Mercy Hospital has given me autonomy, flexibility and support in developing the parish nurse program. The parish nurses are given the same opportunities for creativity and independence. Each nurse sets her work schedule and develops health-education programs according to the congregation's expressed needs. We make an effort to listen to the poor about what they need, following their agendas instead of ours. Four of the parish nurses provide blood pressure screenings and health-education programs at local food pantries. The only limits on this outreach are that the parish nurses do not provide hands-on nursing care nor perform any invasive procedures. We find endless potential for collaboration and resource sharing. The parish nurses show amazing creativity in networking and sharing what does or doesn't work for them.

From January through December 1991, the seven parish nurses made 3,653 client contacts to approximately 1,200 individuals in a variety of environments: office, home, hospital, nursing home, schools, food pantries, personal care homes and other assisted-living arrangements. Two of our most common activities are advocacy and linking individuals, particularly the frail elderly, with appropriate health care and social service agencies. During the first year, providing access to health care was the most significant outcome achieved by our program. Program evaluation consisted of a six-month analysis/reflection by the parish nurses, and a year-end evaluation by the pastors. Congregation evaluations will be completed in the second year.

This past year several of the churches have experienced turmoil and change due to the reassignment/relocation of pastors and the closing and merging of some of the congregations. Through this transition, the parish nurse has been a caring presence whom the parishioners have learned to trust and respect. The professional and non-judgmental attitude of the parish nurse has opened doors that were previously closed and created a trusting environment that allowed spiritual and emotional healing to take place.

The parish nurses grew spiritually and professionally. They support and pray for each other and truly work as a team. Adapting the Dreyfus Model of Skill Acquisition to parish nursing, I have seen the nurses develop from novice to competent and proficient.

I am humbled by God's protection and provision, and amazed at the power of the Holy Spirit as he continues to lead and guide us. We look forward to our second year of serving him and the challenge of expanding the Mercy Parish Nurse

Program through volunteer nurses in additional congregational settings.

Originally published in JCN, Winter, 1993

17

Parish Nursing, Jesus People Style

Norma Singer

Parish nursing conjures up an image of sedate churches and neat, well-tended lawns. Parish nurses are most often associated with suburban churches because city churches cannot afford to pay them even their modest salaries. Some parish nurses do work in the inner city, however, and Maggie Spielman is one of them. Her parish is a homeless shelter on the north side of Chicago near Truman College, called the Cornerstone Community Outreach and run by the Jesus People USA (JPUSA), a part of the Evangelical Covenant denomination. The Jesus People see the shelter as an extension of their church family and treat it as such.

Five years ago Maggie, who holds a master's degree in community health nursing, was in another parish nurse position at Swedish Covenant Hospital. She heard that the hospital was looking for ways to extend their parish nurse program because they wanted to serve the inner city, especially the inner-city poor.

"I was a certified transcultural nurse and really into this cultural thing," said Maggie. "I was drawn to applied anthropology, one of the disciplines foundational to transcultural nursing. I believed that God and values were relative to whatever culture you come from, and as a nurse I wanted to preserve cultures. I wanted to reinforce traditional cultural beliefs to the point where it could be detrimental because the group members may not have decided if they wanted to accept something from the outside or not. At that time, I was opposed to missionaries because I felt they destroyed cultures. I was entrenched in New Age thinking and cultural relativism. Then I met Jesus, and slowly, over the next few years, my worldview completely changed."

Maggie was the first parish nurse the shelter ever had. She quickly realized that the role of the nurse in that situation could encompass all the things a parish nurse does in more traditional settings: integrator of faith and health, health educator, personal health counselor, liaison with congregational and community resources, and health advocate.

"Looking back, I now know that I wasn't a Christian when I took the position, although I believed I was. My hook was the culture. I wanted to study and understand homelessness as a subculture and then provide culturally congruent care. The Jesus People did not ask me what my beliefs were when I interviewed. They may have assumed mine were the same as theirs. They just saw that I wanted to work with homeless people and that I'd done it in the past. They believe God sends them people who need to be there, and I needed to be there. I thought the job would be interesting and cultural, and that's all I wanted. But then, over time, my friends at Jesus People shared the gospel with me, mostly through how they lived their lives and interacted with the homeless people placed in their care.

"At about the same time, another parish nurse invited me to a Bible Study Fellowship group, and that's when I realized that something was missing in my life. One day the teaching leader said that we could pray a prayer of assurance, so I went home and told God I wasn't sure, and I wanted to be sure: I wanted to have a relationship with God through Jesus Christ. Through their actions, my friends had opened my eyes to how authentic Christians live and behave. I became a believer because I saw it lived!" Maggie added enthusiastically.

"This is an amazing place to work because the staff has great fellowship, and we pray with and for our clients. Since I came here, I have never had anyone say no to prayer," Maggie said. The shelter draws people from all over the city, and it is always full. As soon as someone gets housed, more people come. Eighty to ninety people are in the shelter at all times, and Maggie knows every one of them.

"When I come through the door, they start telling me their health woes," she laughed. "We prefer that they come through the centralized system because the Department of Human Services tracks people who are homeless. We have taken people who just show up, but we prefer not to do that.

"One day recently, a couple came to the shelter. The woman was in renal failure—a diabetic on dialysis. We were full, but we made room. The only spot to be found was a storage area. We had been hoping to turn it into a lounge, but we moved everything out and put in some cots, and that's where they're staying. The wife is scheduled for heart surgery next week, and I have had the opportunity to pray with her about that." Maggie's routine changes dramatically when someone like that shows up. Her focus will be on the woman and her husband for a while at least because she'll act as case manager for them.

"Another time we had a mother with developmental delays with several kids who had hernias. In the past she had been unable to schedule and coordinate the pre-surgical work up. We knew that she couldn't handle this situation on her own, so we made it a priority to get the surgeries completed while she lived at the shelter so we could help her."

Prayer is an important part of the shelter's ministry because the staff recognize that the people come because they face crisis on top of crisis. Homelessness is only one part of the crisis they are dealing with. Most are involved in broken family relationships, and prayer is a way to minister to them and help heal family rifts.

Residents of the shelter are mostly women and children and generally live in one big dormitory room on the second floor. However, several rooms on the first floor are available to house intact families or a man and his children. Men are not usually housed, though. The ministry provides three meals a day and helps clients find jobs and more permanent housing. It usually takes at least four months to find housing, harder now that the neighborhood is going upscale. The only affordable places are in bad neighborhoods or in public housing. Gangs make these areas unsafe, but sometimes it's the best they can do.

A woman came to the shelter with five children. One daughter had just returned from visiting her father and had marks and bruises all over her body. "DCFS (Department of Children and Family Services) already has a file on this woman," Maggie said, "and she was upset that they'd think she had abused the girl. I counseled her and helped her think through how she was going to approach this problem. I helped her see that she needed to call DCFS herself. I asked if she'd like me to pray with her before she made the call, and she said yes. We prayed together, and I asked that the truth be known and dealt with. The investigator came to see her at the shelter, and no charges were filed."

Maggie's parish nurse position at the shelter has been funded for five years by Swedish Covenant Hospital. This past year the Michael Reese Foundation provided funding for specific health promotion and primary and secondary prevention programs.

People see Maggie for all kinds of reasons, a common one being public health issues, such as communicable diseases. The shelter does not routinely do blood pressure screenings, but one day a week they run a medical clinic staffed by nurse practitioners, who are sent by a local agency that provides primary care to homeless people. Maggie sees people ahead of time and signs them up for the clinic. She assesses their problems and coordinates all of the details, so they can be handled in an expeditious manner. Then she takes care of the follow-up care, such as picking up prescriptions, distributing them and making sure everyone understands the instructions. People come with the usual complaints: colds, flu, sore throats, sometimes seizures, and always for many prenatal and well-baby exams. The nurse practitioners do the exams, make the diagnoses and write the prescriptions.

"Emergencies are not uncommon at the shelter," Maggie said. "Sue, my Bible study teaching leader, is good at making practical applications of what we are studying. One day she said that rather than come to the Lord with an agenda, we should say, 'Show me what you have for me today.' I distinctly remember the day I prayed that prayer. I was conducting a class with the moms, and they had their kids with them because the day care was full. A new woman came into the group, with her baby wrapped in layers of blankets. He was extremely quiet, but it didn't really concern me.

"Near the end of the class, we were discussing some aspect of HIV, when the woman with the baby said in a timid voice, 'Oh, my baby's been sick, but . . .' and then someone else interrupted her and started talking and talking. When the class ended, everyone needed something. I got so involved with these other concerns that the woman with the baby just disappeared. Something whispered to me (I'm sure it was the Holy Spirit) and said, 'You've got to go find that baby.'

"I went upstairs to the dormitory and found the woman and the baby. After unwrapping the mass of blankets, I took one look at him and knew he was severely dehydrated. We rushed him to Children's Memorial Hospital, and he was admitted for ten days. He could have died! I remember how inundated I'd been that day, with people saying, 'Do this' and 'Do that.' But this quiet, little voice told me to follow up with this woman—and a life was saved. That was the Lord."

The shelter also runs a night program for single women, who are allowed to sleep on mats on the dining room floor because the shelter is a safe place. Sometimes, however, they have to turn women away because they run out of mats.

This is one of the few shelters willing to take teenagers, with their special set of tough problems. When school starts, they try to make sure everyone gets to school.

Spiritual help is always available at the shelter. There's an open invitation to attend the Jesus People's church, which meets in a nearby building each Sunday. "We would never make church attendance mandatory, but we always pray that our witness will make the difference," Maggie said. "The staff talk to each other about God openly before the people around us. We put our faith in Jesus Christ, and we are eager to share the gospel with anyone who is interested."

One of Maggie's closest friends at the shelter, Ginny, was once a homeless woman. She had a ten-year history with the Jesus People and had lived in the shelter twice during those years. Maggie met her several years ago. "Ginny saw how people with Christ in their lives could live, and she accepted him as Savior. She was in a scary apartment on the west side of the city, and she got down on her knees one day and turned it all over to God. Her life was changed. She has been working at the shelter ever since, supervising the night program. Besides having been homeless, she's been a heroin user and on methadone.

"She's an amazing witness to the women who come here at night to sleep, because she's been exactly where they are now. I loved her when she was homeless, and I love her now. She used to have panic attacks and couldn't look you in the eye. She was shaking all the time, and she suffered from severe depression. You'd never know it was the same person. She's living a new life."

The street where the shelter is located is called Murderers' Alley for good reason. Maggie is convinced the shelter has its own swarm of angels protecting it at all times to keep it safe from harm. Only two or three staff people work at night, and the shelter employs no security people.

As part of her ongoing role as health educator, Maggie wrote a grant proposal that has been funded. She has begun teaching American Red Cross classes on first aid and infant and child cardiopulmonary resuscitation (CPR). She's excited because it means the women will learn how to better care for their children, and these new skills could be useful when they go to look for jobs.

Maggie is scheduled to work twenty-four hours a week at the shelter, but she comes as much as she feels she needs to and varies her schedule accordingly. She says she loves her job so much that she'd do it for free.

"I like working here because it's a strong Christian community. We encourage and support each other and are accountable to one another as staff. We need each other. You have to have back up and talk things over with someone when problems arise with residents—they sometimes carry a lot of anger and can be hard to deal with. They lash out, sometimes, screaming and hollering, venting bitterness and vulgarity. It may be directed at other residents, or it may be directed at staff. You have to have someplace to go when that happens, especially when it happens to you.

"Several JPUSA staff members are my accountability partners, and they help me understand and respond appropriately. They may tell me I'm the one who needs to change. We pray together for the Holy Spirit's assistance when that happens because sanctification is an ongoing process for all believers. We rely on God's help in all situations.

"If you're in this work to help people change and expect to see that change while they're here, you'll be disappointed. But we have a heart for the people we are serving, and that seems unique to this shelter. Love makes the difference. Love is the key. Many women who come here have never been loved and, in fact, they have suffered a lot of abuse. They are surrounded by love here. They'll always be able to look back and say that they were cared for by people who were concerned about them as individuals made in the image of God. That's what parish nursing is all about."

Originally published in JCN, Summer, 2001

18

Getting Started
Parish Nursing in a Rural Community

Linda Miles

"For everything there is a season, and a time for every matter under heaven" (Eccles 3:1). My time for parish nursing came in 1994. I was considering a topic for my practicum in advanced nursing practice to fulfill a requirement for my master's in nursing education. When I suggested parish nursing, it was approved.

On a 1992 Christmas card, a friend had mentioned that she was working as a parish nurse. I had no idea what a parish nurse did but was filled with a sense of excitement and curiosity. I wanted to know more about this new nursing role. Although I had worked as a staff nurse, office nurse, school nurse and a director of nurses in long-term care, I was still searching for my niche in nursing.

Getting Started

I contacted the National Parish Nurse Resource Center in Park Ridge, Illinois, and they steered me to their publication *Perspectives in Parish Nursing Practice*. In a section entitled "What's Happening in. . . ." parish nurses from across the country describe what they are doing. I wrote to twenty-two parish nurses; sixteen responded. Enthusiasm and love for the ministries were evident in all the letters. The writers encouraged me to pursue my interest and implement the role in my community.

A review of the nursing literature on the roles of the parish nurse and the church in health care was helpful. Parish nurses are breaking new ground, thus their roles and duties vary widely, depending on the needs of the congregation and/or community. However, all parish nurses function as educators; they address lifestyle issues in the context of Christian values and/or theology.

Underlying this role of educator is the concept of wholeness: the body, mind and spirit are one and cannot be understood as separate from one another. Consistent with Jesus' ministry of healing the whole person, the parish nurse deals with physical ailments, emotional or mental disorders, and spiritual dilemmas. Like Jesus, it doesn't matter what type of brokenness is presented; each person is approached as a whole body. Parish nurses are also counselors, consultants, advocates and liaisons.

The church has been involved in health care since its beginning but over the years has often relinquished physical and aspects of emotional care to the medical profession. Today some church leaders call for the church to reclaim its healing role and to realize it is actually in the field of preventive medicine. The church has information, resources and energy to share with the community. When a parish nurse is added to the church staff, the basic services of the church are expanded from a narrow spiritual focus to include more direct access to health counseling and health education. Nurses and churches make natural partners in holistic care.

My search included the nursing literature on spirituality, spiritual caring and holistic health. Spirituality is different from religion and the psychosocial dimensions of the individual. Professionals have not been able to agree on definitions of spirituality and spiritual caring. Although most nurses believe we have a responsibility to address the spiritual needs of clients, it is often a neglected area of care. When spiritual care is provided, it is often done passively.

An attentiveness to the spirituality of both the nurse and the client is required if parish nurses are to practice holistic care. We cannot be comfortable in dealing with clients' spiritual concerns until we address our own values and belief systems and what gives our life meaning and purpose. Parish nurses must more fully develop the spiritual caring aspect of holistic health so that the spiritual component of individuals can be addressed as systematically as other aspects of client care.

Getting Parish Support

When I met with my pastor, I described the role and responsibilities of parish nurses and my desire to pilot test the rural parish nurse role in our church. We discussed the long-term goal of implementing a community parish nurse project. He was receptive and supportive, and saw a potential for the parish nurse role in our community.

Next, the pastor and elders of the church were informed with written materials about how the concept of parish nursing began. We met and discussed the roles of the parish nurse, the role of the church, benefits for the church and reasons churches and nurses should work together to establish parish nurse programs. The pastor and elders met and approved the pilot project for three months. Meeting with the elders was important; written information alone was not adequate.

I wrote a job description for the parish nurse, identifying principal duties and responsibilities, as well as the required knowledge, skills and abilities. Identifying nursing skills was easy, but I found it more difficult to list the spiritual qualities a parish nurse needs. We set specific goals for the three-month project.

The Pilot Project

I met with the congregation (approximately 25 adults and 19 children), allotting ten minutes to explain the parish nurse role and pilot project. I think more time than this is necessary, perhaps in segments over several weeks, along with handouts and bulletin or church newsletter inserts.

We set four hours a week for parish nurse office hours, and I used my home as the office. Besides the set hours, the congregation was informed that they could call at any time. Most contacts were not during office hours. In a rural community where work schedules are not regular, it is important to be flexible and to let the people know you are available. We notified the local medical clinic about the project, assuring them the parish nurse role did not include any hands-on nursing or duplication of their services.

I regularly attended church functions so I was visible. At the annual meeting, I did a parish health needs assessment. Twenty-eight adults completed the questionnaire, with a separate form for children ages seven to thirteen. Fifty percent of the adults expressed interest in a health program on depression; twenty-one percent said they had had or currently had a mental health problem. The children eagerly expressed health concerns they had about themselves or their families. Everyone was concerned about one particular child. The responses indicated that this child was lacking family support, had poor health habits and low self-esteem.

The three-month pilot project included many other services, such as a monthly health article emphasizing holistic health, blood pressure screenings and teaching a Sunday-school class for preadolescent girls, using Dr. James Dobson's book *Preparing for Adolescence.* I also distributed pamphlets from the American Diabetes Association and the American Heart Association. During Heart Month in February, I created a handout for the children about healthy-heart living that included games and recipes.

As a health counselor, I was often a supportive presence and an active listener. The congregation had concerns about the side effects of medication, health insurance issues and nutrition. Most parishioners contacted me with physical complaints but ended up talking about mental and/or spiritual concerns. One young mother came with her toddler because both had colds. She ended by talking about her need for personal time and the frustrations she was having with her children. Another time a woman came to discuss her medications but talked more about her spiritual needs and how the problems in the world were depressing her. As the clients looked back, they usually noted that they didn't realize when they made the transition from discussing physical to emotional or spiritual issues.

In some situations the parish nurse functions in several roles at once. I have been involved for a few months with a client whose mother is dying of cancer. Before her mother came home from the hospital, I answered her questions and provided information about what was happening to her mother. I referred her to home health for the care her mother needed. She has called me many times to talk, to have questions answered and to receive assurance. I prayed with her for her mother to accept Jesus and went with her twice to pray with her mother. Her mother has accepted Jesus and her impending death. I told her about the hospice program where her mother is now. I continue to support her in prayer and be available when she needs me.

In everything I did, I tried to include the spiritual aspect of health care. Spiritual nurturing contributes to improved life satisfaction and quality of life, improved health, reduced functional disability and lower levels of depression. As people feel better, they are able to reach out to others who are hurting in order to improve their health. Thus, the church's ministry of healing is enhanced. It was difficult to get beyond the stereotype of an RN who provides physical care. It takes time for the holistic approach to be accepted. Parishioners need to see the parish nurses growing spiritually, as well as taking care of themselves physically.

Expanding the Parish Nurse Role

After completing the pilot project, I wanted to expand my role from my parish to the other churches in our small, rural Nebraska town, a farm/ranch community of approximately 800 with seven churches serving the town and surrounding area. The crime rate is low, but there are economic struggles. The population is predominantly elderly, and there seems to be a high rate of depression and cancer. Community clergy are stretched beyond their limits at times to meet the needs of the congregations: the Catholic priest serves three other parishes. My objective was to involve the area clergy as partners in the delivery of spiritual care.

I created and left with the clergy in one-on-one meetings a one-page handout describing myself, defining parish nursing and identifying objectives and activities of the program. I also left with them copies of articles about parish nursing from the winter 1993 *Journal of Christian Nursing*.[1] I was able to meet with five of the six clergy. One had heard Granger Westberg speak, another was aware of parish nurses in his denomination; the others were not aware of the concept at all. All were receptive and expressed various concerns they had regarding the health needs in the community.

Two weeks later I met with the same group at their ministerial association meeting. They viewed the videotape *The Connecting Link*.[2] I answered questions, and we discussed possible approaches to implementing a parish nurse ministry for the community. They committed to spend time during the following few weeks praying and thinking about the implementation of the program.

When they met again, they decided the project should be an individual congregation decision. Each pastor will be meeting with their church leaders and congregations to discuss my proposal. I will be available to meet with church leaders for clarification and to present a program on the role of a parish nurse to the congregations.

What I Learned

To promote a health ministry in a rural community, you need to understand the people in that community: how they think, what they value, the way they live, what they believe and how they communicate. The parish nurse needs to like people. The people need to know that a parish nurse has time to understand and respond to their needs. George Barna reported that one of the keys to an effective ministry is to understand and effectively address people's felt needs.[3] Contemporary Americans are being attracted to churches that clearly communicate a passion for helping people cope with life by providing realistic, practical and caring solutions.

In a rural community parish nurses usually work independently, so networking is essential. Other parish nurses provide encouragement and support, help give direction, share ideas that have worked for them and are a source of spiritual strength.

Originally published in JCN, Winter, 1997

NOTES

1 Janice Striepe, "Reclaiming the Church's Healing Role," *Journal of Christian Nursing* 10, no. 1 (Winter 1993): 4-7 **(in Chap. 3 of this publication)**; Janice Striepe, Jean King and Linda Scott, "Nurses in the Church: Profiles of Caring," *Journal of Christian Nursing* 10, no. 1 (Winter 1993): 8-11 **(in Chap. 14 of this publication)**.

[2] *The Connecting Link*, videotape (Dubuque, IA: The Rural Ministry Program).

[3] George Barna, *The Barna Report 1992-93: An Annual Survey of Lifestyles, Values and Religious Views* (Ventura, Calif.: Regal Books, 1992).

19

Holistic Nursing Care
A Church & University Join Forces

Richard J. Fehring & Marilyn Frenn

Where should people go with health problems related to spiritual distress? What if you were suffering from stress related to an inadequate spiritual outlook? Where can healthy people go for advice on how to stay healthy? Where can physicians send patients with chronic pain related to psychological stress, who didn't want to go to psychiatrists or psychologists?

Our answer is a church-based, nurse-managed wellness resource center.

Several years ago Granger Westberg, a Lutheran minister, proposed that nurses become health ministers in churches.[1] Nurses, he said, could work closely with pastors, identifying parishioners' health needs and providing health promotion services. They could also help people cope with chronic health problems, get into the health care system and care for sick family members in their homes.

Westberg believed churches would be a perfect site for nursing services. Since churches already address spiritual care, they could be bases for holistic nursing care. Ministers are often aware of their parishioners' health needs, and many churches have space available during the week where clinics could be set up. Nurses working with ministers could enhance the services of each.

We had previous experience developing a university-based, nurse-managed center and wanted to develop one at Marquette University's College of Nursing. We knew such centers can offer clients a wide range of services: health education, consultation, screening, assessment, therapeutic relationships and diagnostic management. Since nurse-managed centers are based on nursing models of health care, they also facilitate nursing research and clinical education.

In 1981 there were sixty-four established nurse-managed centers throughout the country and over one hundred in the planning stages.[2] They have been developed in shopping centers, churches, housing projects for the elderly and on university campuses.

Initially we wanted a centralized nurse-managed center at the college with satellite outreach clinics at housing projects, high schools and churches. But our current college building did not have enough space, and we were in the process of moving to a new one.

So in 1981 we wrote a proposal to start with two satellite church-based nursing clinics, one in a Roman Catholic parish and another in a Protestant church. The Wauwatosa Avenue United Methodist Church was interested in expanding its ministry as a "caring, sharing community of faith" and invited us to explain our proposal to its council on ministries.

Building a Dream

The council was receptive to our ideas and voted to go ahead with the proposal. A committee, made up of church members and college faculty, developed plans for a collaborative, ecumenical center. Nine months later, in October 1982, the Wellness Resource Center opened with a health fair presented by our nursing faculty.

The center continues to be governed by a committee composed of faculty, interested church members and the pastor. The committee coordinates publicity, integrates clinic operations with other church programs and serves as a think tank for planning future directions.

The church provided a large room that we divided into space for a small waiting area, private consultation, physical assessment, an area for equipment and client records, and a resource library of books, tapes, biofeedback equipment and a small computer. We use church classrooms for meetings, classes and support groups.

The college and church both contributed equipment, typing and paper supplies, and used furnishings. A Wisconsin United Methodist Foundation, which contributed to ecumenical projects, provided a grant for other equipment and library resources. We request, but do not require, client donations for services.

Faculty, students and community nurse volunteers, most of whom are master's prepared, staff the clinic and provide services like these: health assessment and consultation, health classes, stress management, support groups, community outreach, and screening for blood pressure, cardiac risk factors and diabetes. Community outreach activities have included spiritual well-being assessment at a church fish fry, presentations on stress management, nutrition, exercise and spiritual aspects of wellness to church groups and area public-school teachers.

Clients who come to our Wellness Resource Center complete a self-health assessment based on Gordon's functional health patterns.[3] This assessment tool covers health management, nutrition, elimination, exercise, cognition, sexuality, self-perception, sleep and rest, roles and relationships, coping and stress tolerance, and spiritual values and beliefs. The results of the assessment tool and client discussions with a nurse lead to a nursing diagnosis and plan that includes appropriate referrals.

If medical care is required, we refer clients to their own physician or a physician from our resource file. Several dieticians, social workers and psychologists volunteer their time, so these services are provided at the center.

Developing the Spiritual Dimension

We incorporate the spiritual dimension in a variety of ways. All committee meetings begin with prayer. A minister or priest provides spiritual direction to committee members and to the projects they plan. Clergy also participate in grand rounds and discuss with us how to improve holistic care.

Only qualified nurses work in the center. They must be committed to a Christian, holistic perspective; view health promotion and care of the sick as a ministry; and actively pursue their own spiritual growth through prayer and church activities.

Nurses refer clients to a pastor of their choice for spiritual care but also use spiritual interventions. Relieving suffering and promoting well-being are in themselves ways of providing spiritual care. Also, spiritual assessment is part of each client's holistic evaluation. When a more in-depth spiritual assessment is needed, nurses use a spiritual well-being assessment tool developed by two Christian psychologists.[4] This tool helps clients explore their relationship with God and their purpose and direction in life.

We help clients look at stress from a spiritual perspective and use prayer with our stress management techniques. In teaching relaxation techniques, we encourage clients to focus on their relationship with God rather than repeating nonsensical phrases. Touch and prayer are used when appropriate. However, we never force our spiritual beliefs or practices on clients. Most clients find it refreshing to discuss how spiritual matters relate to their total health.

Another way we attempt to integrate health care and spiritual care is to coordinate clinic services and church activities. Clinic hours coincide with Sunday-morning worship services and with the activities of the church's older adult club. When people see a nurse before or after worship, discussing spiritual health seems to come naturally.

The church has welcomed nurses as health teachers. Nurses, along with the pastor and other members of the church committee, once presented a series titled "Stress Management, Wellness and Coping with Loss." Nurses have taught health classes on Sunday morning and have addressed the men's club, the women's club, the council on ministries and the older-adult club. In addition, they have coordinated two church-based health fairs.

Calculating Success

To evaluate our services, we had our records audited. During the clinic's first two years, it helped 450 clients. Most came for blood pressure testing and maintenance, stress management, diabetic counseling, chronic-pain management or general health consultation.

We reviewed the client's self-health assessments, nursing diagnoses and strategies, and client outcomes. Audit findings showed that we needed to improve our documentation of health teaching, improve our method of scoring the self-health assessments and continue sharing strategies that we each found helpful.

The audit also revealed some gratifying success stories: several people reduced their blood pressure through stress management counseling, biofeedback or meditation. Others sought medical care after discovering their blood pressure was elevated. A boy's frequent nausea and vomiting were significantly relieved after he used biofeedback and imagery. A young man found help in controlling his asthma and discovered a new direction in his spiritual life. An elderly man increased his self-esteem through therapeutic relationships with his nurse and pastor.

The collaborative nature of our Wellness Resource Center has enabled us to project an image of professional nursing that is not evident in medically-oriented practice sites. Individual nurses have reported great satisfaction in their roles, and most of the volunteers have served for over three years.

Students have met both personal and course objectives in the clinic. Undergraduates have participated in blood pressure and risk-factor screening and health fairs as part of their older-adult nursing practicum. One student said this about people at the health fair: "It was really neat because they had so many questions and were so interested in what we were doing."

Graduate students have used the clinic as a practicum for helping clients cope with chronic health problems and have reported great satisfaction with their freedom to develop advanced practice roles. Several graduate students have continued to volunteer time after completing course requirements; one became a member of the governing committee.

The ecumenical nature of our church-based clinic has helped us understand each other's religious traditions and perspectives. So far, we have had Roman Catholic, United Methodist and Lutheran nurses. At a recent healing service, a United Methodist minister and a Roman Catholic lay healer prayed and laid hands on people. Some participants were uncomfortable, while others found the service deeply healing. We have found there are few real problems, as long as we keep Christ central in our relationships and services.

Planning for the Future

We want to continue improving our services. Faculty, students, volunteers and committee members regularly discuss changes and seek God's guidance. Nurses want to work more closely with the pastor and to refer more clients to him. They would also like to try joint interviews where both a nurse and the pastor talk with a client at the same time, and perhaps healing services with the pastor, nurse and client.

Since the Wellness Resource Center opened in 1982, we have started clinics at two housing projects for the elderly and began natural-family-planning services at our school. We are also in the process of developing another church-based clinic in an inner-city Roman Catholic parish.

Located in Milwaukee's poorest district, St. Michael's parish includes Blacks and Hispanics, Laotian and Hmong refugees, and elderly German members. A low-income housing project for the elderly and an urban day-care center are next door to the church. Nurses in the new clinic will visit homebound elderly, assess the health of people in local rooming houses, make home visits with the pastor and help people learn to care for sick family members at home.

We are pleased with our services and are excited about the future. Whether in a suburb or the inner-city, church-based, nurse-managed clinics can facilitate spiritual care, a dimension often missing in otherwise holistic nursing care.

Originally published in JCN, Fall, 1987

NOTES

[1] Granger Westberg, "Dissemination of Wholistic Health Centers." Quoted in O. E. Allen, L. P. Bird and R. Hermann, *Whole-Person Medicine: An International Symposium* (Downers Grove, Ill.: Inter-Varsity Press, 1980), pp. 153-70.

[2] S. Riesch, Nurse-Managed Center Survey, Presentation at First Biennial Nurse-Managed Center Conference. (Milwaukee, Wisc.: June 17, 1982).

[3] M. Gordon, *Nursing Diagnoses: Process and Application* (New York: McGraw-Hill Book Co., 1982), pp. 329-33.

[4] R. Paloutzian, and C. Ellison, "Loneliness, Spiritual Well-Being and Quality of Life." In L. Peplau and D. Perlman, *Loneliness: A Source Book of Current Theory, Research and Therapy* (New York: John Wiley and Sons, 1982), pp. 224-37.

20

Congregational Nurse Practitioner

An Idea Whose Time Has Come

Betty Souther

Congregational Nurse Practitioner! The idea came to me during my first medical mission trip to Mexico along the Rio Grande River with the Baptist River Ministry. I was standing in a poverty-stricken *colonia* along the Texas-Mexico border, helping people who desperately needed basic health care, when the obvious became apparent: why aren't there nurses who have both parish nursing and practitioner skills? What a perfect combination! Why not a Congregational Nurse Practitioner and why not a Missionary Nurse Practitioner?

I had been a nursing instructor at Houston Baptist University (HBU) for over ten years when the school sponsored this first medical mission trip. I was the only nursing faculty who agreed to go. Only then did I learn about sleeping on the floor, taking cold showers and lacking functional toilets. Thirty nursing students, as well as students to run children's ministries and a construction team, made up the mission crew. The spiritual impact of the experience provided the basis for the conception and development of the Congregational Nurse Practitioner (CNP), and potentially the development of a Missionary Nurse Practitioner (MNP) program at HBU.

Family Nurse Practitioners, Pediatric Nurse Practitioners and midwives were becoming established roles, but not Congregational Nurse Practitioners. Why not? If a parish nurse had practitioner skills, as well as spiritual counseling, community development and social service skills, that nurse could be a strong force in the lives of the vulnerable and indigent populations in both rural and urban settings.

Bringing advanced physical and pastoral assessment skills, and in some instances prescriptive authority, to the bedsides of members in a rural congregation could potentially greatly benefit that community. The CNP could link remote sites more efficiently to available physicians and health care resources, as well as spiritual and community resources. Early detection and treatment of spiritual and physical problems can avert a more costly and drastic intervention at a later date.

The focus of the CNP is on the blending of two distinct nursing roles into one unique, innovative role designed to meet the needs of the underserved by using the existing faith community network. This new nurse practitioner role combines the roles of the Family Nurse Practitioner (FNP) and the Congregational Care Nurse (CCN), commonly known as a parish nurse (figure one).

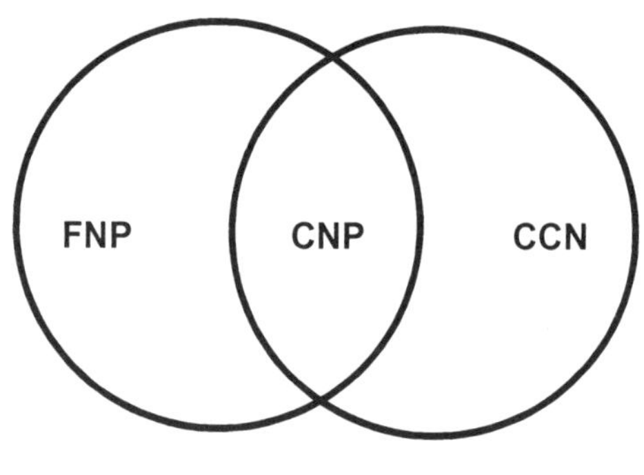

Figure One

Congregation is a more inclusive term that can be used by various denominations, hence we call our parish nurse program Congregational Care Nursing.

The CCN is not an advanced nurse practitioner but is a master of science in nursing degree. In order to offer the innovative Congregational Nurse Practitioner, it is necessary to have both the Family Nurse Practitioner and the Congregational Care Nurse programs.

Currently, the Congregational Care Nurse does not have advanced nursing practice skills but possesses the skills to utilize the faith community network, assess individuals, families, congregations and communities, participate in community development and employ pastoral counseling skills.[1] The CCN has access to the underserved where primary health care is needed but lacks the Family Nurse Practitioner skills to provide that care. Combining the skills of the CCN (parish nurse) with that of an FNP into the new role of Congregational Nurse Practitioner would transform the nurse into a powerful instrument for the delivery of spiritual and primary health care.

The faith community is a natural network and support system that provides access to people across the life span, ethnic groups, denominations and socioeconomic levels.[2] Churches have existing facilities, a system of formal and informal networking in the community, a grasp of the human needs of their congregations and the community's trust. The existence of social networks and social support through the faith community provides the nurse the mechanism through which the unmet spiritual, health and human service needs of the underserved individuals, families, aggregates, communities and societies (IFACS) can be addressed.

The CNP and the CCN can provide health care to IFACS where the traditional health care delivery system is unable or unwilling. Clearly, a nurse who has the skills of an FNP combined with the knowledge of congregational care and faith community resources can affect the health of the underserved.

Two underserved populations that have an affinity for the faith community are the Hispanics and the elderly. Many of these groups live in large urban areas served by multiple primary, secondary and tertiary care centers, but because of lack of insurance or other resources, they have difficulty accessing these facilities. In Texas, many of the underserved populations live in the rural areas, but because of lack of personal resources or lack of health care practitioners, they have limited access to health care. Rural hospitals in Texas are closing every year due to lack of financial assets, triggered by the inability of the underserved populations to afford traditional fee-for-service care.

The size of Texas produces unique problems that other more densely populated states do not face.[3] Additionally, the proximity of Texas to Mexico, coupled with the poor Mexican economy and the impossibility of patroling the extensive border, has made Texas an attractive refuge for the Mexican people. Currently it is estimated that 550,000 illegal Mexican immigrants contribute $290 million to the economy but cost $456 million in health care, educational and prison services.

When looking at a map of the Texas counties that need physicians, it can be said that "where the grass doesn't grow, the docs don't go!" The remarkable point is that most of the counties that need physicians have an abundance of churches. Approximately 60% of the Texas counties have five or fewer physicians; frequently one might find only two physicians and twenty churches. Noteworthy is the high percentage of the counties' population who are church adherents, suggesting the importance of the role of the church in the lives of the people in medically underserved counties. Why not use the churches as an outreach to the community of need?

The Hispanic and elderly populations have traditionally had strong ties to the faith community. In Texas the Hispanic population will access the church and church-related facilities before attempting access to the traditional health care system, especially if that facility is government-supported. The Hispanic community in Texas has a distrust of government institutions, particularly if the Hispanic individual is illegal.

The expanding Hispanic population has far-reaching effects for the United States that we must begin to acknowledge and address through our actions and not merely with well-meaning talk. The U.S. Census Bureau figures project Hispanics only a few years away from becoming the largest ethnic minority in the country.[4] Projections indicate that Hispanics will tie African Americans at 12.4 percent by the year 2005. By the year 2050 the Hispanic population is projected to reach 22.5 percent of the U.S. population. In Texas the Hispanic population grew 24.3 percent from 1980 to 1990.

Due to uncontrolled border crossings and the climbing average age of the population, the Hispanic population produces health needs that burden the existing health care system in Texas and will begin to affect other parts of the nation. Soon not only states like Texas, California and New Mexico will be straining to find resources to cope with the problem, but other states as well will be affected because of migratory patterns of the illegal workers and the aging of our people. Clearly we must address the issue of providing health care access to Hispanics and the elderly, as well as meeting their economic, social and spiritual needs.

No nurse practitioner programs that prepare the graduate for a congregation-based practice exist in the U.S. In Texas ten schools produce Family Nurse Practitioners, educated to provide underserved health care through clinics, hospitals or other health care settings. Practice based on the needs of a specific faith community or group of communities can potentially serve a greater number of the population.

The Congregational Nurse Practitioner program as implemented by Houston Baptist University has many unique, cutting-edge qualities. The CNP will serve the vulnerable and indigent populations of Texas through church outreach programs, pastoral counseling skills and community development skills. The concepts taught in the program will be geared for both urban and rural needs and will be generic to congregational nursing throughout the U.S. While currently fewer than five programs nation-wide offer master's degrees in parish nursing, only the program offered by HBU will offer a blend of the roles of the Family Nurse Practitioner and the parish nurse.

Both the CNP and the CCN will take courses from our master's of arts in psychology and pastoral counseling (MAPPC) degree program. The CNP and the CCN may earn the MAPPC degree by taking twenty-four to twenty-seven additional semester hours.

In the future I hope that we will be able to answer the need beyond our state, extending into the foreign mission field. I visualize the Congregational Nurse Practitioner as the home missionary nurse and the Missionary Nurse Practitioner as the foreign-based missionary nurse. Currently it is difficult to find physicians willing to give their lives to the mission field. I believe there are many nurses who would be willing to serve God as medical missionaries.

In many of the areas where foreign missions operate, high-tech, sophisticated medical care is lacking. Physicians in these areas practice traditional, low-tech, hands-on medicine, using available resources and their own wit.

Most of the skills needed in these areas are within the scope of practice of the Family Nurse Practitioner, so why not develop the Missionary Nurse Practitioner to serve these areas? He or she could easily fill some of these pressing needs overseas.

With a seminary located on HBU's campus, I believe we should develop a curriculum encompassing FNP skills and congregational skills, and be able to obtain the missionary prerequisites. Once the Congregational Nurse Practitioner program is fully developed and accepted by the faith community, we will implement the Missionary Nurse Practitioner program.

Originally published in JCN, Winter, 1997

NOTES

1 Sandra Bergquist and Judith King, "Parish Nursing: A Conceptual Framework," *Journal of Holistic Nursing* 12 (1994): 155-70.

2 Jan Striepe, "Reclaiming the Church's Healing Role," *Journal of Christian Nursing* 10, no. 1 (Winter 1993): 4-7 **(in Chap. 3 of this publication).**

3 Tim Lopes, "Hispanic Muscle Going Unflexed: Lobbyists Also Prove Ineffective for a Divided Community," *The Houston Chronicle* (April 16, 1995).

4 U. S. Bureau of Statistics, "Statistical Abstract of the United States 1994: The National Data Book" (1996).

21

Beyond Band-Aids™ *Empowering a Honduran Community to Care*

Nancy J. Crigger & Lygia Holcomb

Tegucigalpa, the capital of Honduras, is an earth-colored quilt of ochre, sienna and gray on approach from the air. Once earthbound, reality shapes the quilt into houses and buildings of a Third-World city. The 600,000 city dwellers, like many who live in underdeveloped countries, suffer poverty, addiction, crime, disease and death. Our health care team of six nursing students, four registered nurses (including one nurse practitioner), a pre-med student and a physician brought supplies, teaching programs and expanded clinic services to a community church, the *El Centro Evangelico Vida Eterna* (CEVE). We hoped to alleviate a small portion of the suffering that is commonplace in Tegucigalpa.

After a few days in the clinic setting, the team members discovered that our episodic Band-Aid™ approach to health care, based on the medical model, was not the most beneficial for this community.[1] We concluded that only an ongoing health care program that involved community members would result in lasting changes in the health status of the people. We felt a program based loosely on the parish nurse model could augment the medical model currently used at CEVE.

What Led to the Trip

Since the University of Central Florida, the school where we taught, had been in the process of internationalizing their curriculum, we were motivated to develop a course in which students would deliver health care to vulnerable and underserved populations. A representative from a church in West Palm Beach, Florida, had contacted us about CEVE in Honduras, and we had begun planning a week-long mission. Since the university is a secular institution, the team volunteers had various religious beliefs, but many were motivated by Christian commitment to serve others.

People Served

Three social strata exist in Honduras: the Hondurans of European descent, who are the educated and wealthy; the Miskitos or cowboys, who are descendants of indigenous people, like the Mayans; and the black Garifuna people, whose descendants came from Africa. The Garifuna have historically occupied the coastal areas but recently have moved into urban areas such as Tegucigalpa.[2] Migration of other national or cultural groups has occurred, especially from neighboring Central American countries and Asia. The social boundaries among the diverse groups within the city are blurring, but distinctions are still evident.

Women's status in Honduras is low. The poor women often lack education, bear a large number of children and rarely are given the opportunity to rise above their station. The cost of a marriage license is prohibitive for many of the poorer women. The church, without legal sanctions, marries some couples, while others just live together. Without legal marriages, fathers may abandon the women and children without fear of retribution. Then mothers become the sole supporters of their children. If they are unable to provide for the children, become ill or die, the children may become homeless.

From what we observed, the women have little choice but to remain in a relationship, despite the cultural male behavior pattern of sex outside of marriage (prostitutes and mistresses) or other forms of mistreatment. Families are large, especially in the rural areas, with the fertility rate of almost five children per woman. Sixty-two percent of Hondurans earn less than $60.00 (U.S.) per month.[3]

The Resources

Education for Hondurans of the lower socioeconomic class is limited. Public schooling is offered through the fourth grade, with an additional four years if the student is a high achiever. School is not mandatory or free. The cost of uniforms prohibits attendance for many children. College and professional education are all but impossible for the poor in Honduras. Literacy rates hover around 50 percent overall, even lower in the rural areas.[4] TVs are common in many homes, even of the very poor, but educational programming is minimal.

The government provides health care for the indigent in clinics and hospitals. But they are usually overcrowded, requiring an average five-hour wait, and are run by Honduran physicians in training or volunteers. The clinics are underfunded and overwhelmed with the health needs of the community. AIDS (*SIDA* in Spanish) is a severe and growing problem in Honduras. The government has an HIV program that focuses on prevention, but people with HIV/AIDS are simply not treated.[5]

Infection and vermin plague the poor of Tegucigalpa. Poor hygiene and nutritional deficiency[6] compound the environmental maladies. Mortality among children under five is high at 111 of 1000.[7] Many people die of preventable diseases because of poor or nonexistent health care. Common causes of death are respiratory or diarrhea episodes leading to dehydration complicated by malnutrition.[8] Women die from AIDS, cancer and complications of pregnancy and childbirth.[9]

The Church Community

CEVE is housed in a small building, constructed by the church members. Their goal is to raise the level of well-being of the community. The church leadership and members believe that their ministry is to help the poor help themselves by education (learning a skill) and by offering a health clinic alternative to the government health care system. Dr. Daniel is an elder of CEVE and also the physician-director for the small, church-supported clinic. The doctor, assisted by his wife, has daily office hours in the clinic and also makes home visits in the community. He bases his practice on disease prevention and health promotion. Unknown to us, the doctor was out of medicine and had asked God for a sign if he should continue his work in this church. When we arrived and filled the pharmacy with donated drugs and the clinic with patients, he praised God for the miracle and answer to his prayer.

Our health care team worked closely with Dr. Daniel. Using additional space in the church, we saw seventy-five to one hundred people a day, but we turned away many more who sought services. The number seeking health care was just too great. We also held classes on health-promoting behaviors, and the sanctuary filled with people anxious to learn.

The church membership is highly varied—professional people, nurses, lawyers and teachers, as well as lower-income Hondurans who come from other neighborhoods within the city. CEVE serves four groups: the poorer church members and constituency, the street kids and people who live under the bridge, the river people and the women and children of the brothel district.

One church member, who lived close to the church and helped prepare our meals each day, had diabetes. She knew diabetics should not eat sugar but did not have equipment or knowledge to test her blood level. She reported that she never put sugar in her coffee, but each day at lunch she drank an orange soda loaded with sugar. We supplied the clinic with glucometers and instructions for testing blood sugar, but what was needed was an extensive diabetic education program.

The street kids and bridge people live on the downtown streets and under a bridge near the downtown area. Often these people are either addicted to drugs or are from the rural areas and unable to find work and lack the resources to return home. The street kids and bridge people have no recourse but to beg or steal to exist. We often saw children accept partially-consumed colas or half-eaten food from strangers or grab leftover food from plates in open-air restaurants, as diners left their tables. The thirty to fifty street kids to whom the church ministers are all (without exception) addicted to glue. The longer children are on the street, the more likely they are to become glue sniffers.[10] The kids get so high on the glue that some use marijuana to sleep. We saw abandoned children as young as six years old. We spoke to one little boy who was so young when he was forced into the street that he did not know his age.

Most of the street children are male, but there are a few girls. They often become pregnant. No government agencies step in to protect the children, so they and their babies remain homeless. I remember one homeless teen who was twenty-eight weeks pregnant when she came to the clinic but had only gained three pounds during her pregnancy. A diet history revealed that she had eaten one sandwich in the last two days. She had obviously sniffed glue recently; glue was on her clothes and hands. A nursing student asked her what would convince her to stop using the glue. The teen replied, "Getting off the streets." She felt that if she had a home and people who cared about her, she could get along without the high from the glue.

Two Christian men have an ongoing ministry to these children and provide sandwiches several times a week for them. They also bring the kids and bridge people to the clinic and to CEVE services and events. These children are filthy, ill and vulnerable to injury and disease. The kids, however, try to help each other. We saw three street boys helping one of the young mothers carry her child, who was ill, several miles to the clinic.

The river people live in the immediate vicinity of the church. They are generally uneducated and live marginally on income from some type of work, such as making or selling tortillas on a street corner. Large numbers of people live in connected one-room shacks with dirt floors near a highly polluted river. Many bathe and wash clothes in the river. Children play in it. Human and animal waste pours into the river. Most of the shacks have no running water or waste disposal. Even in this malaria-endemic country, the windows are open holes without screens. The dusty dirt roads between the shacks are filled with bare-footed children and thin, mangy dogs. Health problems abound, and the level of understanding of illness prevention seems to be low. The people were hospitable and let us into their homes and brought their families and neighbors to the church clinic and health education sessions. One man even invited us to a special dinner where he barbecued one of his goats for us to enjoy.

The red-light district of Tegucigalpa is about a twenty-minute drive from the church. Many of the women came from large, poor families and began prostitution in their early teens. Uneducated and young, they felt they had little choice except to become prostitutes. Most of the women are HIV positive, and many of their children also have HIV. We took a large number of condoms with us to distribute to these women, but they refused them, stating that the men would not use them. Our experience contradicts the 1993 study by Laura Fox and her colleagues that about 75 percent used condoms.[11]

One prostitute had a history of galactorrhea of two-years' duration, not associated with pregnancy or lactation. She had not seen a physician but had lived with the condition, knowing something was wrong but not trusting the public health care system enough to seek medical attention. She was upset about her problem, and without the slightest hesitation, showed me her breasts and the profuse galactorrhea. The biggest concern for a woman with this symptom is pituitary tumor. I was shocked that the condition had been untreated for so long. I discussed the need for further diagnostic tests with Dr. Daniel.

The women conduct business and live with their children in the brothels. They are housed in one-room windowless cells. Our health care service had to begin after the women awoke in the afternoon and end by 4 p.m. so the women could begin prostitution. Conditions within the brothel were horrible, and it is no wonder that more seriously ill children were seen there. One brothel owner let us use his personal bedroom for examining the families, and we held several clinics there. The children were pale and quiet. They had fevers, skin infections with cellulitis, parasitic gastrointestinal illness and malnutrition. Their mothers had multiple health problems such as diabetes, hypertension, respiratory illness, gastrointestinal pain, chronic headaches and evidence of physical abuse.

Strangely, the first patient I saw in the brothel was a man dressed as a woman. He was the transvestite lover of the brothel owner and had a respiratory illness complicated by AIDS. He was very trusting that I could help him. He even told me his male name for our records. I gave him antibiotics and some vitamins, but I explained that he needed much more treatment. He was grateful that I had taken time to see him. I spent a few minutes discussing nutrition and safer sex practices, and a minister prayed with him. Once again we were only able to see a fraction of those who sought health care, and our vitamins, antibiotics and worm medicine were insignificant in the face of the health needs.

CEVE members are committed to providing services for the four populations they have been led to serve, but they also want to change conditions. They saw the needs of these people and the void of resources within the community and rose to intervene. Their philosophy for intervention is to use three important resources—spiritual growth, education and health care to help others help themselves. They bring many strengths to the community: a commitment to vulnerable, underserved populations; the ability to use available resources; sensitivity; and the ability to network. They are committed to helping the poorest of the poor. They love and accept the poor, the ill and the outsider. They bring them into their buildings, even those who are filthy and high on drugs. They seek these vulnerable people out in the brothels and on the streets.

The CEVE members are remarkably creative in using available resources. They built their church brick by brick, as they could afford each addition. They are culturally sensitive. For example, the minister asked a nurse to cook our food while we were there, believing that her knowledge of sanitation would keep us from becoming ill. Translators were always provided for us.

The CEVE members also network. They have established ongoing exchanges with churches for ministry in the U.S. CEVE members are negotiating with the brothel owners for ways to help the women learn new skills to support themselves and their children.

As the first U.S. health care team to visit the church, we were encouraged to see that the populations to whom CEVE members minister are receptive to participating in health care and health education. However, it was obvious that episodic visits of a U.S. team were inadequate to address the health needs of this community.

Set within the philosophy of the church's framework and from our experiences, our role shifted from episodic health care to planning and implementing an ongoing preventive program that would teach and reinforce positive health behaviors. Long-range goals include changes in public policy that would provide sufficient sanitation, safe food, clean water and air, and a safe environment for all community inhabitants. The immediate purpose of the program is to improve the health status of women and children in the populations the church currently serves.

A Nursing Practice Model

Parish nursing is a fitting framework for developing a practice model for our church community philosophically and practically.[12] Parish nursing promotes health care with the spiritual dimension for individual healing and well-being. The philosophy of parish nursing and of this church promote individual independence and responsibility.[13] Practically, one physician is incapable of meeting the overwhelming health care needs of the community without additional trained personnel to assist him. Drawing on the existing strengths of the church and the willingness of community members and others to participate, it seems that parish nursing could provide much needed assistance to the doctor and improve the health of the community. Although parish nursing may sometimes be limited to the church community, the members of CEVE also are dedicated to providing care for the poor whom God has called them to serve. Therefore, our model addresses health outreach, as well as the needs of the church members. Parish nursing speaks to the three broad elements of a practice: structure, process and values.[14] Although the three elements are related—for example, values affect the structure and process—each can be discussed separately.

The Structure

The limited number of professional nurses in the church community meant we had to plan to train lay members of the church as health workers. The health promotion ministry will be directed by a trained nurse, who is responsible to the minister and the physician who head the clinic (see figure below). An advisory board with representatives from each of the four populations will assist the director and the health promoters in appropriately assessing and intervening in the community.

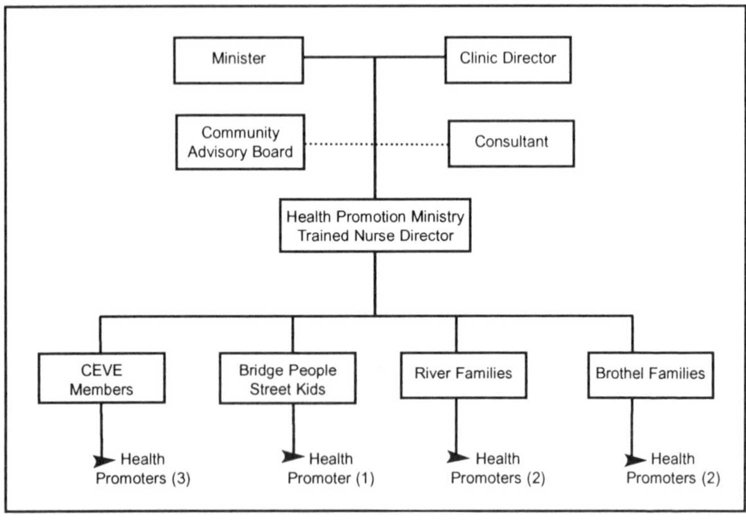

Practice Model for CEVE Community Church

Our role in the development and implementation of the health promotion ministry will be to plan and implement two curricula, one for the director and one for the health promoters. Once the ministry is implemented, we will provide additional education or consultation as needed. Electronic mail, which is available through the church, makes communication between the U.S. consultants and the health promotion ministry readily accessible. Members of a local Florida church frequently travel to CEVE and are willing to transport educational materials.

Those in the health promotion ministry program will be Honduran nurses and lay volunteers from the church. Volunteer health promoters will initially be trained to teach health promotion, to do health assessment and to assist in the treatment of minor health problems. Each health promoter will be assigned to one of the four populations of the church ministry.

The Process

The director of the health promotion ministry team will be responsible for communicating with the church staff and will work in conjunction with the minister and the physician. The director of the health promoters will work closely with the consultants and the advisory board. The director is responsible for specific duties and assignments for the health promoters and for their ongoing educational support. The director will call and chair regular meetings of the health promotion ministry.

Women volunteers from the church will be selected for training as health promoters. They will not replace the current clinic-based program but augment it. Suggested criteria for selecting these women include having lived in the community, spiritual maturity, good verbal and written communication skills, and time and willingness to learn and to work.

The health promoter will make home visits in the community or meet with clients at a designated location. She will also work with groups of women and children in the community. The health promoter will be educated to serve in four capacities: educator, referral source, nurturer and health monitor.[15]

As educator, the health promoter will teach individuals and families about making positive health choices that will result in behaviors that prevent disease and improve health. Education will focus on providing facts and health information, but the health promoter will also assist people in applying the information to their own life situations. Initially, the health promoters will concentrate on teaching about nutrition, hygiene and reducing environmental hazards to health.

The health promoters will refer clients for health care to the church clinic or to public facilities for treatment of illness, immunization and health screening. Then the physician will be able to concentrate on the care of those who have medical needs. Although few public assistance programs are available in Tegucigalpa, by networking the health promoter may locate other resources. For example, she could refer someone without job skills to the church job training programs.

The health promoter nurtures through maximizing the well-being of women and children and CEVE's community in general. Well-being includes physical, spiritual and mental health. The health promoter may minister to the spiritual needs of the client or may refer the individual to appropriate counseling or spiritual resources within the church. For many people in these vulnerable populations, merely seeing someone who cares enough to visit and touch them improves their sense of self-worth and brings hope.

Last, but equally important, is the health promoter's role as a health monitor. She will go to homes or living areas and assess health status. She will record growth and development of children, assess potential health hazards in the environment and help women and independent children to problem-solve about ways to reduce these hazards, and monitor illness prevention such as immunization and cancer screening. In collaboration with the doctor and program director, the health promoter may provide follow-up monitoring of recovery from illness and control of chronic health disorders. She may measure blood sugar and blood pressure or assess wound healing in between visits to the physician. She will manage problems within her scope of training such as control of lice and scabies, treatment of minor injuries and encouragement of health-promoting self-care. The health promoter will also provide ongoing assessment of her assigned community.

The Values

Designing a curriculum to be used for any group of students that are as culturally and educationally diverse as the health promoters is a major challenge. One must not only explore the best teaching-learning process but also the content appropriateness within the curriculum and the difficulty that non-native language speakers have in effective communication.[16] The curriculum is in the process of development but will contain ethical and health care related concepts.

The ethical concepts that underlie the health promotion ministry program are *agape* and *autonomy*. *Agape* is Christian love that is not fondness or passion but rather a willingness to act in good will for the benefit of another.[17] *Agape* love is extended unconditionally for human existence and not because of any qualities possessed by the recipient.[18] This love is permanent and stable. *Agape* in our philosophy and curriculum is the extension of good will toward another that is evidenced by unconditional acts of good will.

Autonomy is also an important ethical concept that applies to the church community. The uneducated and poor within that body are often socialized to assume a dependent role in their health care and in many other aspects of their lives. By preparing community members to make positive health care choices and to engage in health promoting behaviors, the decision maker becomes more autonomous and empowered.

The goal of the health promotion ministry is to enhance and promote spiritual, mental and physical health; to care for minor health problems; and to refer problems requiring more extensive treatment. The long-range goal of the health promotion ministry is to empower the community to make lasting changes that benefit the well-being of all community members.

Originally published in JCN, Winter, 2000

NOTES

1 Cheryl Larson, "Parish Nursing: Caring for the Whole Person Within a Church Community," *ISN Bulletin* (1995).

2 Guillermo Yuscaran, *The Garifuna Story*, 2nd ed. (Tegucigalpa, Honduras: Nuevo Sol Publications, 1997).

[3] Basic Socioeconomic Data (March 16, 1998), available at http://database.iadb.org/INT/BRPTNET/english/hndbrpt.htm.

[4] Alison Acker, *Honduras: The Making of a Banana Republic* (Toronto: Between the Lines, 1988).

[5] Catherine O. Keeffe, "Confronting the Stigma of AIDS," *Nursing Times* 90 (1994): 35; Laura J. Fox, Patricia E. Bailey, Kuzu L. Clarke-Martinez and others, "Condom Use Among High-risk Women in Honduras: Evaluation of an AIDS Prevention Program," *AIDS Education and Prevention* 5, no. 1 (1993): 1-10.

[6] Isabelle Romieu, Mauricio Hernandez-Avila, Juan A. Rivera and others, "Dietary Studies in Countries Experiencing a Health Transition: Mexico and Central America," *American Journal of Clinical Nutrition* 65, supplement (1997): 1159s-65s.

[7] World Vision, 1997, available at http://www.worldvision.co.nz/ohonduras.html.

[8] Ann V. Millard, "A Causal Model of High Rates of Child Mortality," *Social Science and Medicine* 38, no. 2 (1994): 253-68.

[9] Pan American Health Organization, 1996, available at http://www.paho.org/english/ honduras.htm.

[10] Martha C. Wittig, James D. Wright and Donald C. Kaminsky, "Substance Use Among Street Children in Honduras," *Substance Use/Misuse* 32, no. 12 (1997): 805-27.

[11] Fox, Bailey, Clarke-Martinez and others: 1-10.

[12] Lois J. Coldewey, "Parish Nursing: A System Approach," *Health Progress* 74, no. 9 (1993): 54-57; Joan K. Magilvy and Nancy J. Brown, "Parish Nursing: Advanced Practice Nursing Model for Healthier Communities," *Advanced Practice Quarterly* 2, no. 4 (1997): 67-72.

[13] Larson, "Parish Nursing: Caring for the Whole Person".

[14] Nancy Hoffart and Cynthia Q. Woods, "Elements of a Nursing Professional Practice Model," *Journal of Professional Nursing* 12, no. 6 (1996): 354-64.

[15] Granger Westberg, "A Historical Perspective: Holistic Health and the Parish Nurse," in *Parish Nursing: The Developing Practice*, eds. Phyllis A. Solari-Twadell, Anne M. Djupe and Mary A. McDermott (Park Ridge, Ill.: National Parish Nurse Res. Ctr., 1990), pp. 27-39.

[16] Lois Frels, Jeanette Scott and Mary A. Schramm, "A Process: Development of a Model Multiculturalism Curriculum Designed for

Mobility Across Geographic Borders," *AANA Journal* 65, no. 4 (1997): 339-45.

[17] Gene H. Outka, *Agape: An Ethical Analysis* (New Haven: Yale University Press, 1972).

[18] Soren Kierkegaard, *Works of Love* (originally 1847, reprint New York: Harper & Row, 1962).

Part Five

Spiritual Care

22

Spiritual Care
Assessment & Intervention

Linda L. Treloar

Spiritual concerns fall toward the bottom of the priority scale in most health care settings. Many nurses avoid spiritual issues, believing that they will experience censure or lose their jobs if they provide spiritual care. In an attempt to protect the patient from proselytizing, hospital policies often prohibit considerations of religion by staff members. Is it any wonder that health professionals experience confusion and fear and avoid integration of spirituality into health care?

Spirituality has no universally accepted definition or meaning in the nursing literature.[1] Some describe the spirit as the *life principle* at the center of our being, integrating and transcending the biological and psychosocial nature. They see spirituality as a "basic or inherent quality in all humans that involves a belief in something greater than the self and a faith that positively affirms life."[2] According to Pamela Reed, spirituality involves the making of meaning through relatedness to dimensions that transcend the individual in a way that empowers but does not devalue the individual.[3] Spirituality involves the search for meaning and existential purpose in life in relation to self, community (others), environment (nature) and a higher being.[4] Definitions of spirituality may involve horizontal (humanistic) or vertical (religious) dimensions. However, spirituality is applicable to all persons, whether religious, humanistic, atheistic or agnostic.[5]

An emphasis on the wholeness of life is not new. *Holy, whole* and *heal* are derived from the same root word. Religion and health have historical connections in most cultures. Physician-priests during biblical times and religious monastic orders during the Middle Ages indicate an enduring concern with the wholeness of life by both religion and health professions.

Florence Nightingale recognized that spirituality is intrinsic to human nature and is our deepest and most potent resource for healing.[6] However, Nightingale's work represents a split between nursing as a spiritual calling, represented by the lady with the lamp, and that of a science/profession, represented by the sanitary engineer.[7] Science replaced nursing's religious roots during the age of rationalism. Today the public has begun to recognize the limitations of the scientific worldview: everything is not measurable, and the mind and spirit influence healing. Health is seen not as the absence of disease but in the sense of wholeness or well-being. Theologian Jürgen Moltman writes: "True health is the strength to live, the strength to suffer and the strength to die. Health is not a condition of my body; it is the power of my soul to cope with the varying condition of that body."[8]

Why Isn't Spiritual Care Given?

Spirituality is only minimally integrated into health care for a number of reasons: (1) An empiricist influence on Western medicine, in which only the tangible, material and measurable is real, is incompatible with spirituality. (2) Consistent with this, limited nursing theory has been developed relative to spirituality. (3) Not all agree that nurses can and should give spiritual care. (4) Separation of church and state as applied to spirituality and health care practice is misunderstood.

(5) Nurses feel inadequately prepared to provide spiritual care. A 1990 national survey indicated that 97 percent of 186 practicing RNs believed that nurses should address patients' spiritual needs, but only 66 percent felt prepared to do so.[9] (6) Spiritual needs may be mistaken for psychosocial needs. (7) Personal embarrassment, discomfort with one's own spirituality and the belief that spirituality is a private matter are other restraining factors for many nurses. (8) Finally, some believe that spirituality should be limited to chaplains and clergy.

Yet patients want health care providers to be involved in spirituality. In Dana King and Bruce Bushwick's study of 203 inpatients, 77 percent said that physicians should consider patients' spiritual needs, although 68 percent said their physicians never discussed religious beliefs with them. Nearly half (48%) wanted their physicians to pray with them.[10] In Reed's study of 300 adults, 27 percent listed "arranging a visit with clergy" as the most frequent spiritual intervention.[11] Timothy Daaleman and Donald Nease found that patients' frequency of religious service attendance (at least monthly) predicted their acceptance of physician inquiry into their spiritual/religious practices and acceptance of referral to pastoral staff.[12] Assessing the frequency of religious service attendance provides one easy measure for receptivity to discussion about spiritual concerns.

Both professional and regulatory bodies encourage integration of spiritual care considerations into health care practice, but we lack guidelines for practice. The 1973 International Council of Nurses Code for Nurses says: "The nurse, in providing care, promotes an environment in which the values, customs and spiritual beliefs of the individual are respected."[13]

The NCLEX Practical Nurse Test Plan states that the practical nurse collects data regarding spiritual needs of the client and assists in planning measures to provide spiritual support. The NCLEX Registered Nurse Test Plan specifies that the registered nurse uses knowledge, skills and abilities that include but are not limited to religious and spiritual influences on health. Various accrediting bodies, including the Joint Commission on Accreditation of Hospitals and Organizations (JCAHO), The National Hospice Organization and Medicare, require that spiritual needs of clients be addressed.[14]

Multiple studies demonstrate a positive association of well-being, health, social support and financial status with intrinsic religious commitment and organized religious activities.[15] Spiritual beliefs provide feelings of hope, well-being and strength to live with chronic illness.[16] Prayer and other religious activities are commonly used as coping strategies.[17]

Integration of spiritual caregiving into nursing practice involves several areas of emphasis. Nurse scholars must participate in concept development and research. We must teach students and health professionals how to promote spiritual health by openly discussing these concepts, in conjunction with demonstration and modeling. Every nurse must assimilate spirituality into practice; the depth and breadth of spiritual interventions will reflect the nurse's spiritual maturity.

Assessment for spiritual distress and spiritual well-being begins with two basic nursing diagnoses: *spiritual distress* and *potential for enhanced spiritual well-being.* Outcomes of spiritual therapeutics for the patient/family include: (1) recognizing inner strengths, purpose and meaning of life, feelings of hope; (2) perceiving harmony with self, others, God and the environment; (3) stress reduction, or even healing. The key areas for assessment include: (1) general and personal spiritual beliefs, (2) identification with a specific religion, (3) spiritual or religious support systems and rituals, (4) spiritual distress or an opportunity for enhanced well-being.

Since spiritual growth may be limited by psychosocial and cognitive development, assessment in children calls for a different approach. Children need to be reassured that God loves and accepts them unconditionally, forgives them and never abandons them. They may exhibit spiritual distress behaviorally through withdrawal, anger, disrupted sleep, crying, repeated questions or by regressed or resistant behavior.

All nurses can and should assess for spiritual needs in patients and family members. Nurse practitioners and other advanced practice nurses are in an ideal position to integrate spirituality into health care practice and to model this for other health care professionals and allied health staff. Taking a comprehensive health history in addition to focused health assessments provides opportunities for assessment of a patient's spiritual health status. Providing care on a continuing basis to patients at end of life or with life-threatening illness usually increases the prominence of spiritual care issues.[18] Situations that create distress, whether physical, emotional or cognitive, usually increase spiritual care needs for patients and their families. At these times, spiritual health needs may be the most obvious, most urgent and most readily amenable to alleviation, *if they are recognized and appropriate intervention follows.*

Spiritual Assessment in Children

1. How do you feel and who or what do you turn to when you re in trouble, when you re scared?

2. Tell me about any church or religious activities that you or your family participate in.

3. Can you tell me about God? Can you draw a picture of you and God?

Assessment Questions

A nurse may ask the patient or family such questions as:

1. What gives your life purpose and meaning? What/who is the source of your strength and hope? What is your concept of God or a Supreme Being?

2. What are your thoughts about your health in relations to your spiritual beliefs?

3. How has illness affected the way you view yourself?

4. How have you coped in the past through times of difficulty or pain? What religious rituals or practices are important to you?

5. How has this situation affected your thoughts about God/Supreme Being or the practice of your faith?

6. At the end of life, are there things you want to do or people you need to speak with? What unfinished business remains? Do you want to forgive anyone or seek forgiveness?

Any nurse, religious or not, should respect a patient's or family's right to follow personal religious practices. Usually this requires that the nurse initiate direct conversation with the patient/family about these issues: "How can I help you to carry out your faith/beliefs?" Nurses can promote the expression of spirituality in the patient/family by creating a climate that communicates love, value and worth, and that respects others' cultures, beliefs and practices related to health and illness. This means that nurses are aware of personal values, biases and myths, and are comfortable with their own spirituality. The nurse must listen with both heart and ears.

Linda Ross's data suggest that nurses who gave spiritual care at a deep level were aware of the spiritual dimension in their own lives, having experienced personal crises causing growth.[19] I believe that my ability to relate to others facing serious or chronic illness reflects my lived experience and personal spiritual growth as the parent of a young adult disabled with neuromuscular disease.

How Shall We Intervene?

Spiritual care interventions include the use of religious materials (e.g. Scripture reading); the opportunity for prayer and meditation, music/singing and attendance at spiritual services; and referral to clergy, support groups or parish nurse programs sponsored by local churches. Prayer may be offered as an adjunct to medical treatment. Rarely will a patient/family be offended by the question: "May I pray for you?" Basic to determining the appropriateness of use of prayer is the question, *Whose needs will be met: mine or those of the patient/family? What would the patient/family pray if he/she were to do so?*

My students often tell me they're uncomfortable with the idea of praying for someone. I reassure them that their awareness of these feelings is useful, and that praying for another requires comfort with one's own spirituality. Other students ask, "How will I know what to pray for? What if the patient asks to be healed of his disease?" Asking the patient/family what their hopes are and what concerns they would like addressed through prayer is the first step. Before I pray, I silently ask that God will use me to help meet the person's spiritual needs. Restating the hopes, concerns and fears that the patient/family shared and requesting comfort and support of the patient/family is very useful. God is not a magic genie. While physical healing may result from prayers of faith, it is not guaranteed.

Do nurses actually pray for patients? How well do they implement spiritual care strategies? In a study of 303 Christian nurses, 35 percent initiated conversations about spiritual matters at least weekly with patients, 43 percent with colleagues/peers. Seventeen percent of these nurses made offers to pray with patients at least weekly, 21 percent offered to pray with colleagues/peers. Integration of self-reported Christian beliefs and values into nursing practice and greater comfort in providing spiritual care increased with age.[20] My personal experience supports this: as I have grown in my faith, I have become more comfortable with meeting the spiritual needs of others.

As a geriatric/adult nurse practitioner, I routinely ask patients and their families, "Is faith or a religion important to you?" Often the spiritual or religious perspective of older adults is visible in their environment. I commonly find a Bible, a religious wall hanging, plaque or picture of Jesus. Then it is easy to say, "I notice you have a Scripture verse on your wall (or a Bible on your table). Do you have a faith or religion that is important to you? Knowing this information will help me to plan care with you that reflects your beliefs and wishes." I ask whether there is clergy contact or opportunities for participation in religious rituals, and if the patient's spiritual/religious needs are being met satisfactorily.

If I am unable to get this information from the patient, I ask the patient's family. No one has become upset when I inquired about spiritual beliefs and/or religious faith. The discussion of advanced directives for medical decisions usually involves consideration of spiritual and religious beliefs. If no interest is shown in spiritual issues, my assessment goes no further, unless spiritual distress is evident. Usually the patients and their families are delighted that I asked them about their spiritual beliefs.

As I have grown in maturity as a health professional and in my own spiritual life, discussion of spiritual issues and provision of spiritual care that meets the patient's and the family's needs has become easier. Occasionally I offer prayer, and the patient and family often thank me and tell me they feel comforted. But when I teach students and health professionals about spirituality and giving spiritual care, I often hear, "I don't have time."

Not long ago one of my students required supervision during the administration of IV narcotic analgesia to a patient recently diagnosed with metastatic lung cancer. The student told me the patient was struggling with her grave diagnosis and had been crying. She remarked that she felt helpless to relieve the woman's distress. When I entered the room, I suggested the student sit at the patient's bedside while giving the pain medication. I noticed a Bible on the patient's bedstand, and brightly colored hand-drawn children's pictures adorned the walls of her hospital room. I remarked about the patient's Bible and asked if she had a religious faith that was important to her. The patient quickly affirmed this. I then asked if a pastor or clergy had offered to visit. She responded that she was not having any visitors other than her immediate family because she couldn't deal with people's questions about her condition.

She began to cry and immediately complained that she had asked on two previous days for a hospital chaplain to be called, but no one had come. I asked what she had expected the chaplain to do for her. She said she wanted prayer. Her tears flowed. I offered to pray for her, and she consented. I prayed for comfort and strength for her and her family, for wisdom for her and the health care staff and for future decisions about treatment. When I finished, she reported a great sense of comfort.

Afterward I helped the student to make certain that the staff requested a visit by the chaplain. I suspect that it had simply been forgotten. How much time did this spiritual care intervention require? It began during the administration of narcotic analgesia and took ten minutes. Spiritual care can often be incorporated into everyday interactions with patients, requiring no extra time.

Integration of spiritual care into practice seems to be related to perception of spiritual need and to personal beliefs and values.[21] We can expose nurses to basic spiritual assessment and intervention strategies, but maturity appears to promote a higher level of intervention.[22] Spiritually mature Christian nurses are ideally suited to role modeling for students and other staff. Spirituality is an integral part of health and the whole person. Research demonstrates positive benefits of religious or spiritual activities on health outcomes. The purpose of considering spirituality in health care is to create an environment that promotes rather than inhibits the spiritual expression of patients and their families. It is the responsibility of every nurse.[23]

Originally published in JCN, Spring, 1999

NOTES

1 Thom J. Mansen, "The Spiritual Dimension of Individuals: Conceptual Development," *Nursing Diagnosis* 4, no. 4 (1993): 140-47.

2 Mary Ann Miller, "Culture, Spirituality and Women's Health," *Journal of Obstetric, Gynecologic and Neonatal Nursing* 24, no. 3 (1995): 257.

3 Pamela G. Reed, "An Emerging Paradigm for the Investigation of Spirituality in Nursing," *Research in Nursing and Health* 15 (1992): 349-57.

4 Margaret A. Burkhardt and Mary Gail Nagai-Jacobson, "Reawakening Spirit in Clinical Practice," *Journal of Holistic Nursing* 12, no. 1 (1994): 9-21; Lynda Juall Carpenito, *Nursing Diagnosis: Application to Clinical Practice,* 6th ed. (Philadelphia: J. B. Lippincott, 1995).

5 Verna Benner Carson, *Spiritual Dimensions of Nursing Practice* (Philadelphia: Saunders, 1989); Elizabeth J. Forbes, "Spirituality, Aging and the Community-Dwelling Caregiver and Care Recipient," *Geriatric Nursing* 15, no. 6 (1994): 297-302; Nancy C. Goddard, "Spirituality as Integrative Energy: A Philosophical Analysis as Requisite Precursor to Holistic Nursing Practice," *Journal of Advanced Nursing* 22 (1995): 808-15; Gertrude K. McFarland and Elizabeth A. McFarlane, *Nursing Diagnosis and Intervention: Planning for Patient Care,* 3rd ed. (St. Louis: Mosby, 1997).

6 Janet Macrae, "Nightingale's Spiritual Philosophy and Its Significance for Modern Nursing," *Image: Journal of Nursing Scholarship* 27, no. 1 (1995): 8-10.

7 Barbara Stevens Barnum, *Spirituality in Nursing: From Traditional to New Age* (New York: Springer, 1996).

8 Jürgen Moltmann, "The Liberation and Acceptance of the Handicapped," in *The Power of the Powerless* (San Francisco: Harper & Row, 1983), p. 142.

9 Carolyn Kresse Murray, "Addressing Your Patient's Spiritual Needs," *American Journal of Nursing* 95, no. 11 (1995): 16N, 160-61.

10 Dana E. King and Bruce Bushwick, "Beliefs and Attitudes of Hospital Inpatients About Faith Healing and Prayer," *The Journal of Family Practice* 39, no. 4 (1994): 349-52.

11 Pamela G. Reed, "Preferences for Spiritually Related Nursing Interventions Among Terminally Ill and Nonterminally Ill Hospitalized Adults and Well Adults," *Applied Nursing Research* 4, no. 3 (1991): 122-28.

12 Timothy P. Daaleman and Donald E. Nease, "Patient Attitudes Regarding Physician Inquiry into Spiritual and Religious Issues," *The Journal of Family Practice* 39, no. 6 (1994): 564-68.

13 Alice Pappas, "Ethical Issues," in *Nursing Today: Transitions and Trends,* 2nd ed. J. Zerwekh & J. Claborn, eds. (Philadelphia: W. B. Saunders, 1997), p. 363.

[14] James R. Dudley, Cheryl Smith and Martin B. Millison, "Unfinished Business: Assessing the Spiritual Needs of Hospice Clients," *The American Journal of Hospice & Palliative Care* (March/April 1995): 30-37.

[15] Harold G. Koenig, *Aging and God: Spiritual Pathways to Mental Health in Midlife and Later Years* (New York: Haworth Pastoral Press, 1994); Charles Marwick, "Should Physicians Prescribe Prayer for Health? Spiritual Aspects of Well-Being Considered," *Journal of the American Medical Association* 273, no. 20 (1995): 1561-62; Barbara M. Dossey and Larry Dossey, "Body-Mind-Spirit: Attending to Holistic Care," *American Journal of Nursing* 98, no. 8 (1998): 35-38.

[16] Cathy Young, "Spirituality and the Chronically Ill Christian Elderly," *Geriatric Nursing* 14, no. 6 (1993): 298-303; Verna Benner Carson and Harry Green, "Spiritual Well-Being: A Predictor of Hardiness in Patients with Acquired Immunodeficiency Syndrome," *Journal of Professional Nursing* 8, no. 4 (1992): 209-20; Verna Carson et al., "Hope and Spiritual Well-Being: Essentials for Living with AIDS," *Perspectives in Psychiatric Care* 26, no. 2 (1990): 28-34; Jacqueline Ruth Mickley, Karen Soeken and Anne Belcher, "Spiritual Well-Being, Religiousness and Hope Among Women with Breast Cancer," *Image: Journal of Nursing Scholarship* 24, no. 4 (1992): 267-72.

[17] Patricia E. Camp, "Having Faith: Experiencing Coronary Artery Bypass Grafting," *Journal of Cardiovascular Nursing* 10, no. 3 (1996): 55-64; Theresa L. Saudia, Marguerite R. Kinney and Leslie Young-Ward, "Health Locus of Control and Helpfulness of Prayer," *Heart & Lung* 20, no. 1 (1991): 60-65; Kathy E. Sodestrom and Ida M. Martinson, "Patients' Spiritual Coping Strategies: A Study of Nurse and Patient Perspectives," *Oncology Nursing Forum* 14, no. 2 (1987): 41-46.

[18] Arlene Stepnick and Tess Perry, "Preventing Spiritual Distress in the Dying Client," *Journal of Psychosocial Nursing* 30, no. 1 (1992): 17-24.

[19] Linda A. Ross, "Spiritual Aspects of Nursing," *Journal of Advanced Nursing* 19 (1994): 439-47.

[20] Carolyn Hall and Hilreth Lanig, "Spiritual Caring Behaviors as Reported by Christian Nurses," *Western Journal of Nursing Research* 15, no. 6 (1993): 730-41.

[21] Ross, "Spiritual Aspects," 439-47.

[22] Hall and Lanig, "Spiritual Caring Behaviors," 730-41.

[23] Judith Allen Shelly and Sharon Fish, *Spiritual Care: The Nurse's Role*, 3rd ed. (Downers Grove, Ill.: InterVarsity Press, 1988).

23

Spiritual Assessment
Comparing the Tools

Rosemarie A. Vandenbrink

Puzzles. I find them time consuming and frustrating, as each piece is unique in shape, color and position. Yet, perhaps God doesn't share my views on puzzles. Several years ago, I heard the analogy that God's plan is a puzzle, and every person is a piece in that puzzle; moreover, God's picture would be unfinished without me.[1] God knows where I belong in his puzzle.

Throughout each day, I have endless opportunities to cooperate with the hand of the Creator, as he molds and colors my small puzzle piece to fit into his design. By saying yes to his vision of me, I help him complete his puzzle. This paradox prompted me to rethink situations and circumstances. This insight has been instrumental in my spiritual growth, has given me solace during difficult times, has changed how I view life and has engendered my holistic view of health. As a result, I now view health and wellness as a puzzle. Each of us is unique, with our physical, psychological, social and spiritual dimensions intertwined. Each aspect of this dynamic network supports and strengthens us in our journey of life.

A person's spirit is manifested in either an empowering or destructive way throughout life. The present turbulence in our society may be the natural result of viewing the spiritual as a low priority. One's spirit is the source of his or her vision. The spirit synthesizes life's events, giving us meaning and purpose. Time to ponder in silence is hampered by radios, televisions, Walkmans,™ computers and other activities that call out to us. With little opportunity for reflection, we neglect the spirit, and our well-being becomes seriously affected. Disease and morass result. It is plausible, then, that some of the maladies we face are symptoms of a spiritual need.

So, how can we assess this elusive aspect of health? What tools are available for me to assist clients toward holistic health and wellness? Are these tools useful in establishing a nursing diagnosis related to spirituality? I explored these questions during my three-month practicum at Redeemer Evangelical Lutheran Church in London, Ontario, Canada.

For the practice of parish nursing, few tools existed in the nursing literature developed by and for nurses. I searched for reliable, convenient tools that would assess the spiritual well-being of parishioners and address the reciprocal nature of each piece in the puzzle of health and wellness. I decided the JAREL Spiritual Well-Being Scale[2] and Ruth Stoll's Guidelines for Spiritual Assessment[3] were the most relevant for this area of nursing and had the most promise for answering the questions I posed. These tools assessed well-being in relation to faith practices, beliefs, relationships and communication. I decided to compare these two spiritual assessment tools, since each would use a different approach to assess the parishioner's perceived emotional, spiritual, social and physical wellness. The JAREL Spiritual Well-Being Scale is a Likert scale scored after its completion, whereas Stoll's Guidelines for Spiritual Assessment are open-ended questions.

The parishioners volunteered, after encouragement, to participate in the evaluation of these tools in two ways. They agreed to complete one, with or without my assistance. I developed questions to critique the assessment tools, and the participants also completed this questionnaire. I received excellent feedback from both tools that enabled me to assess the spiritual health of the parishioners who participated in my study.

The JAREL Scale was the easiest and fastest assessment tool (figure one below); it assessed the present internal resources used in coping with life's situations. However, many parishioners experienced difficulty in choosing an option on the Likert scale, with the wording of certain questions and the meaning of specific concepts (such as *spiritual well-being* and *afterlife*) seeming unclear to them. Further, a parishioner's vision, hearing or other communication impairments such as expressive aphasia or the presence of depression, stress and anger also affected the completion of the scale. Nonetheless, these parishioners would not have been able to answer or complete Stoll's open-ended questions either.

Stoll's Guidelines required much reflection and a considerable amount of time to complete. However, richer data were obtained. Parishioners noted this assessment was "a solitary instrument to be done alone in one's chamber" where "with no distractions, one can proceed at one's own pace and concentrate better." The assessment "provided an opportunity to re-examine my relationship with God"; it "felt like I'd been on a spiritual retreat all by myself." One parishioner aptly concluded, "I'm not sure my circles would have encompassed the same items tomorrow." Life experiences, age, education, health, solitude and time affect one's recollection. The spiritual assessment enlightened the parishioners' understanding of who they were at that moment.

A nursing diagnosis of spiritual distress or enhanced spiritual well-being could be established from either assessment tool. Introspection focused on spiritual well-being created knowledge by clarifying feelings, beliefs and actions. Parishioners were able to see the connection between thought and action, between knowledge and values and how their physical, emotional and social well-being mirrored their spiritual wellness. When I assisted a parishioner with either assessment tool, our discussions encouraged self-examination, which defined terms and resulted in a more detailed response and self-awareness. Our conversation elucidated strengths, personal resources, coping mechanisms and, subsequently, problems or concerns.

For the parishioners who were not able to think quickly or on the spot, being given time to ponder concepts like *spiritual well-being* and *afterlife* prior to completing the assessment would have been beneficial. Both tools facilitated empowerment and

JAREL Spiritual Well-Being Scale

Directions: Please circle the choice that best describes how much you agree with each statement. Circle only one answer for each statement. There is no wrong answer.

	Strongly Agree	Moderately Agree	Agree	Disagree	Moderately Disagree	Strongly Disagree
1. Prayer is an important part of my life.	SA	MA	A	D	MD	SD
2. I believe I have spiritual well-being.	SA	MA	A	D	MD	SD
3. As I grow older, I find myself more tolerant of others' beliefs.	SA	MA	A	D	MD	SD
4. I find meaning and purpose in my life.	SA	MA	A	D	MD	SD
5. I feel there is a close relationship between my spiritual beliefs and what I do.	SA	MA	A	D	MD	SD
6. I believe in an afterlife.	SA	MA	A	D	MD	SD
7. When I am sick, I have less spiritual well-being.	SA	MA	A	D	MD	SD
8. I believe in a supreme power.	SA	MA	A	D	MD	SD
9. I am able to receive and give love to others.	SA	MA	A	D	MD	SD
10. I am satisfied with my life.	SA	MA	A	D	MD	SD
11. I set goals for myself.	SA	MA	A	D	MD	SD
12. God has little meaning in my life.	SA	MA	A	D	MD	SD
13. I am satisfied with the way I am using my abilities.	SA	MA	A	D	MD	SD
14. Prayer does not help me in making decisions.	SA	MA	A	D	MD	SD
15. I am able to appreciate differences in others.	SA	MA	A	D	MD	SD
16. I am pretty well put together.	SA	MA	A	D	MD	SD
17. I prefer that others make decisions for me.	SA	MA	A	D	MD	SD
18. I find it hard to forgive others.	SA	MA	A	D	MD	SD
19. I accept life situations.	SA	MA	A	D	MD	SD

Figure 1

growth by addressing relationships, encouraging thought and molding care specific to the parishioner's season in life.

To enhance spiritual well-being and feelings of being connected, focused nursing interventions could be implemented with the scored results of the JAREL Scale and with the responses to Stoll's assessment guide. Further, Stoll's questions could be used as an adjunct to the JAREL scale.

Stoll's Guidelines for Spiritual Assessment

Concept of God or Deity

1. Is religion or God significant to you? If yes, can you describe how?
2. Is prayer helpful to you? What happens when you pray?
3. Does a God or deity function in your personal life? If yes, can you describe how?
4. How would you describe your God or what you worship?

Sources of Hope and Strength

1. Who is the most important person to you?
2. To whom do you turn when you need help? Are they available?
3. In what ways do they help?
4. What is your source of strength and hope?
5. What helps you the most when you feel afraid or need special help?

Religious Practices

1. Do you feel your faith (or religion) is helpful to you? If yes, would you tell me how?
2. Are there any religious practices that are important to you?
3. Has being sick made any difference in your practice of praying? In your religious practices?
4. What religious books or symbols are helpful to you?

Relations Between Spiritual Beliefs and Health

1. What has bothered you the most about being sick (or in what is happening to you)?
2. What do you think is going to happen to you?
3. Has being sick (or what has happened to you) made any difference in your feelings about God or the practice of your faith?
4. Is there anything that is especially frightening or meaningful to you now?

Excerpted from Ruth I. Stoll, "Guidelines for Spiritual Assessment," American Journal of Nursing, September 1979, pp. 1574-77. Used with permission.

Figure 2

Other interventions could be prayer, reading, music, helping someone less fortunate, spending time with a child or a loved one, and/or attending a religious ceremony or cultural event. Furthermore, a clergy visit could be suggested and encouraged.

Our spirit is a dynamic force that enables us to feel linked with our inner being, with others, with our families, with our communities and, ultimately, with God. The relationship between spiritual beliefs, health and illness should be explored. As wellness advocates, our passion for holistic health drives us to investigate pragmatic ways to elucidate the real needs of our clients. The insights enable us to provide the necessary care and support. Moreover, sensitivity to the possible spiritual root of a problem results in effective caring interventions.

A spiritual assessment may be the first step in opening the doors of one's heart and mind to Christ. Reflection synthesizes thoughts, feelings, situations and circumstances. A person's spirit is able to reframe an uncontrollable situation with choices. With these choices we can realize some power.

For example, suffering can be viewed as merely tragic or as an opportunity to find our place in the puzzle of life. Illness and other hardships have meaning and purpose, if seen as an opportunity to say yes in the ongoing creation of our own puzzle piece and ultimately of the Lord's full picture. Nursing is a visual sign of empathy, warmth, love and hope, if our care validates feelings and reaffirms our client's value and potential within God's larger picture.

A nurse's integrity and care foster an environment of trust, where spirituality can be expressed and where clients feel heard and respected. Honest, open introspection that looks deep into one's mind and heart is the essence of a spiritual assessment. The process of comprehending ourselves as a work-in-progress can be frustrating and time-consuming.

However, these are the essential elements of health promotion and of personal growth. A person's spirit provides dynamic internal resources that touch every aspect of his or her being. Each of us is uniquely shaped and created to fit perfectly into God's master puzzle. We do not stand in isolation but are supported by and connected to others and to God.

Assessing this rudiment of health is an edifying activity that emphasizes that there are no schisms in a person's wellness. It has a strong potential to elicit harmony of body, mind and spirit in the life of the participant and an emancipatory potential that must be respected and utilized. The synergy of body, mind and spirit is crucial to health and wellness. Spiritual assessment is not a perfunctory exercise but a vital tool to foster holistic health and excellence in nursing.

Originally published in JCN, Summer, 2001

NOTES

1 R. Scallon, "Say Yes," *Say Yes*, Dana, Heartbeat Music HBC 9.

2 JoAnn Hungelmann et al., "Focus on Spiritual Well-Being: Harmonious Interconnectedness of Mind-Body-Spirit—Use of the JAREL Spiritual Well-Being Scale," *Geriatric Nursing* 17, no. 6 (1996): 262-66.

3 Ruth I. Stoll, "Guidelines for Spiritual Assessment," *American Journal of Nursing* 79, no. 9 (September 1979): 1574-77.

24

Spiritual Care
How the Christian Community Cared for Mama

Luberta D. McDonald

After years of meeting my patients' spiritual needs, I met an unexpected challenge. My ninety-one-year-old mother was diagnosed with pancreatic and stomach cancer. Two and a half weeks later, she died. Mom knew God. She had a vital prayer life. When Mama prayed, God answered—and everybody knew it. She read her Bible throughout each day, and God spoke to her. A former school-teacher, she never lost her zest for learning about God and the world.

Six months earlier I had moved home from Atlanta to a little house across the street to be near her in my hometown, Adel, Georgia. Although she appeared to be in good health, she seemed more frail, and I suspected she would soon need my help and support. Several months after I'd moved, she phoned at 6 a.m. saying, "I'm sick, and I need you to come." When I arrived, she was cool and clammy, with a pulse of forty. I called an ambulance to transport her to the hospital. During her hospitalization she was diagnosed with diverticulosis, anemia and bradycardia.

After returning home, her weight and appetite steadily declined. Further testing revealed pancreatic and stomach cancer. Several days later, she asked me if anything could be done. I said, "No, nothing can be done at this point."

She nodded her head and said, "Okay. I can accept it."

Mama was a strong woman who had always cared for others. Now it was her turn to be supported. She began to reach out to others. She asked her friend, Yvonne, to read the Bible to her. I realized my mother needed spiritual care. Spiritual care involves a systematic assessment of a patient's spiritual needs, followed by a care plan with appropriate interventions. According to Judith Shelly, "A spiritual need is anything required to establish and maintain a dynamic, personal relationship with God."[1] Spiritual care includes such interventions as worship, compassionate presence, prayer, Bible reading, devotional literature, human touch, music and the love and support of the faith community.

Bible Reading

My mother loved to read, especially the Bible. Before she became bedridden, she would sit and read for hours. She persisted even as her vision failed because of glaucoma. I tried to ensure that the area was well lit, and she had her primary reading materials at her fingertips. Friends gave her large-print Bibles to read. She also found a large-print devotional book.

Psalm 37 particularly brought her comfort. "Trust in the Lord, and do good; so you will live in the land, and enjoy security. Take delight in the Lord, and he will give you the desires of your heart. Commit your way to the Lord; trust in him, and he will act" (Ps 37:3-5). "I have been young, and now am old, yet I have not seen the righteous forsaken or their children begging bread. They are ever giving liberally and lending, and their children become a blessing" (Ps 37:25-26). These verses expressed her hopes, dreams and experience with God.

Worship

Mama and I talked openly about her death. She didn't seem afraid. She planned carefully. I told her I would like to sing at her funeral and asked which song she preferred. "You don't have to try to do that," she replied, aware of the strain that would put on me. "I want to," I assured her. Mom loved to hear me sing, and I wanted to honor her.

A few days passed, and she named the song, "The Lord Is My Shepherd." Sitting by her bed, I asked if she wanted me to sing it for her then. With a quiet smile, she said, "Yes, that would be good." I sang the song I would sing at her funeral. "The Lord is my Shepherd, I shall not want. He maketh me to lie down in green pastures. He leadeth me, he leadeth me beside the still waters. He restoreth, he restoreth my soul. Yea, though I walk through the valley of the shadow of death, I will fear no evil, for thou, for thou, art with me. . . . Surely, goodness and mercy shall follow me, and I will dwell in the house of the Lord, forever and ever." As I sang, Mama worshiped God, as she echoed the words and raised her hand in praise. This memory will be forever etched in my heart and mind.

Faith Community

My mother loved her church; she was a devoted member. She especially loved the pastor and his wife. She served as the church's secretary for over fifty years. One day she asked me to calculate the last time she attended church. She hated to miss. The pastor and his wife visited and gave her Communion. They gently and carefully helped her sit up to receive the elements. Mother seemed to deeply appreciate the visit.

After learning of the severity of Mama's illness, the pastor came by regularly, visiting and praying with her. During his visits she felt comfortable enough to share her deepest concerns, and even to cry (something she rarely did with anyone else).

Prayer

Other pastor friends visited and prayed for her. Reverend Ensley recalls Mama asking why the Lord had not yet come for her. He told her, "You have a purpose for being here."

She asked, "What can I do, just lying here?" He said that she was a silent witness. She accepted this. He visited often and offered her comfort. He sat close to her bedside, held her hand and spoke quietly and lovingly to her.

Human Touch

Often as I, or other visitors, sat at her bedside, she communicated by extending her hand. As her energy decreased, she communicated primarily through touch. An affectionate woman, she knew the value of loving human touch. As I sat on her bed one day, I put my arms around her as she lay there. I caressed her, as we expressed our appreciation of each other. I listened intently to her every word, as though it would be her last. She said, "Thank you for being so kind to me."

"You are welcome, Mama," I replied. "I wouldn't want it any other way."

Music

One day when Mama had become much less communicative, our friend, Alex, visited. Instead of talking, he sang. He knew of Mom's pilgrimage of faith and encouraged her through his singing and by reading the Bible to her.

According to Ruth Folta, "Not only can singing provide diversion and modify attitudes and emotions, but it can also be relaxing and releasing. Therapists tell us that it is most beneficial, initially, to find music that is similar to the patient's present mood and progress from there."[2] Alex, sensitive to mother's serene mood, quietly sang and read to her. Her body language communicated peace and relaxation.

Faith Community

Many people came to visit Mama. I tried to accommodate each as best I could. They seemed so appreciative of her and just wanted to be near her. Several of my friends traveled long distances when they heard she was dying. They wanted to see her at least one more time. The love and support of the church and community overwhelmed us. The people came, and we felt loved. As Mom grew weaker, I sometimes had to turn people away. It was hard for many to accept the fact that she was dying.

Shelly states, "Illness changes a person's status in the worshiping community. When people can no longer attend worship services and church functions, they may quickly become isolated from the rest of the congregation."[3] It is vital to develop creative ways for the patient to remain involved in their faith community. Visits help to keep the homebound patient connected to the faith community, relieving isolation.

Compassionate Presence

Spiritual care includes care for a patient's family. Fortunately, most of the hospice personnel assigned to our family shared our faith. The nurse seemed comfortable sharing her faith with us. She took cues from what I shared and from our environment. Bibles, pictures of Jesus and Christian plaques were all around our home. She said she assesses each patient and family to know how to best provide spiritual care. She recognized that people have various faiths.

I remember when the nurse first asked me how I was doing with my mother's illness. Although it was her job to assess the caregiver, I appreciated her sensitivity. Her attentive and unhurried approach, as she asked questions and listened to me, put me at ease. She was kind to my mother and me. She clearly communicated compassionate presence. It helped to ease the process of Mom's terminal illness and death for both my mother and me.

Compassionate presence includes listening, spending undisturbed time, patience, attentiveness and sensitivity that lead to appropriate interventions, or merely being with another person. This is probably the most important gift we can offer another person.

Physical Care

As Mama's illness progressed, I began to care for her physical needs. The first time I bathed Mom was a deeply spiritual experience. I had not given a bed bath in years. I wanted to be gentle and show her respect. In my mind, I envisioned what it would be like to allow Jesus to give this bath through me. As I began with this goal in mind, gentle care flowed into my mind and actions. I experienced Jesus' presence, giving her bath through me. I will never forget this encounter with Jesus and with my mom. It was such a gift to extend dignity, gentleness and honor to one so needy. Jesus said, " . . . just as you did it to one of the least of these who are members of my family, you did it to me" (Mt 25:40).

Why Give Spiritual Care?

Although exhausting and draining at times, caring for my mother was a deeply satisfying experience. The spiritual care that the hospice nurse and our faith community provided gave both my mother and me strength and encouragement. As nurses, we have the opportunity to bring the same comfort and spiritual support to others.

Originally published in JCN, Fall, 2000

NOTES

1 Judith Allen Shelly, *Spiritual Care: A Guide for Caregivers* (Downers Grove, Ill.: InterVarsity Press, 2000), p. 29.

2 Ruth H. Folta, "Music: Arousing the Human Spirit," *Journal of Christian Nursing* 10, no. 2 (Spring 1993): 29.

3 Shelly, *Spiritual Care: A Guide*, p. 60.

25

Spiritual Care
Reflecting God's Love to Children

Betsy Anderson & Sue Steen

How do we get started giving spiritual care to our patients? The basis of all nursing care is the nursing process. Spiritual care of children and families begins with nursing assessment. Knowledge of the child's and the family's faith routines gives the nurse helpful ways to offer support during a child's hospitalization.

Within the context of a family, a child learns about health and illness, right and wrong, life and death, and faith in God. Families are instrumental in teaching children major belief and value systems for life. Therefore, spiritual care for children cannot be provided without considering the whole family.

In caring for children, the needs of the family are a major focus. During a crisis, children easily sense fear and anxiety in their parents. If parents are supported in their coping efforts, children are better able to handle the ups and downs of hospitalization. Parents are better able to support their child if nurses provide adequate information and incorporate them into the child's care. A child's spiritual needs are always easier to understand after assessing the parents' spiritual needs.[1]

A relationship of trust and open communication builds bridges to children and creates the environment in which a child or parent can reveal deep thoughts, concerns and spiritual struggles. Spiritual assessment of both the child and family is important. A nurse can build trust with children by talking first with parents. This can ease the child's fears and increase the likelihood that children will share their amazing life insights with us.

Faith has different meanings for different people. For Christians, faith is most often a stable, hope-giving support system. However, for other people, talking about faith may intensify guilt or feelings of bitterness. We must respect a person's right not to talk with us about spiritual issues.

As nurses, we also must be sensitive to the rights of parents to influence their children in the spiritual dimension. This does not mean, however, that we can ignore faith or spiritual issues. We must be ready and willing to talk with children and families about spiritual issues at any time. After we assess each situation, we then will be able to provide sensitive spiritual care based on the identified needs without pushing our own faith agenda.

Nursing has acknowledged the importance of a spiritual dimension, but few nurses have been taught how to systematically assess spiritual needs. As is true with all nursing care, spiritual care interventions must be based on objective assessment data. According to Judith Still, dangers in using intuition alone in determining spiritual needs include bringing our own experience or perspective to the patient's unique situation and the danger of unconsciously meeting our own needs instead of the patient's needs.[2] Subtle intuitions must be validated by the child and family. We must understand the child's or family's situation before prematurely intervening.

How Do We Assess Spiritual Needs?

Making a spiritual assessment of a child and family consists of gathering background information, making careful observations and taking a faith history. Understanding the normal fears and concerns of children at various developmental levels provides the nurse with a comfortable, natural starting point. Seven-year-old Jessica told her nurse that she got cancer because she hit her brother. When the nurse explored this with her, Jessica stated that God was mad at her for being mean to her brother.

Background information on religious affiliation is collected from most patients on admission to the health care system. Denominational affiliation alone does not provide information on whether faith in God is an important source of help and strength. Neither does a lack of identified religious affiliation necessarily mean a family is uninterested in spiritual issues. This information is important, however, as a starting point for spiritual assessment.

Routine observations of behavior, verbalizations, the environment and the child's significant relationships give the nurse clues to the importance of faith to a family. Observable cues can easily be gathered before a nurse probes more deeply into spiritual issues.[3]

Hospitalization often creates fear and anxiety in children. They may use stalling techniques, have nightmares or demonstrate regression. Lonely children may misbehave, become uncooperative or withdraw. The nurse must continually listen for and inquire about feelings or misconceptions behind a child's behavior. Parents are especially helpful in observing their child's subtle behavior changes and helping professionals understand what the child is telling us through this behavior.

A parent's behavior also gives important clues to spiritual needs. When faced with a life-threatening diagnosis, parents may blame themselves for not recognizing their child's signs and symptoms earlier. Spiritual needs may be expressed through behavior such as anxiety, hostility and blaming.

Routine daily activities incorporated into a child's care are also clues to the importance of faith and religion to the child and family. Prayer before meals or bedtime provide consistency with home routines for some young children. This can be comforting to a hospitalized child. Dietary restrictions also may point to the importance of religious practices in a family's life.

Reflection on what a child or family member frequently verbalizes provides helpful information. For example, does the child talk about church or church activities? Does the family mention God? Is the parent asking questions about why tragic events happen? When a child frequently talks about the death of a pet, he may be reflecting fears about death or spiritual distress. The child's environment can reveal evidence of a faith life. Bible storybooks at a child's bedside provide an opportunity for the nurse to talk with the child about spiritual things. Cards, gifts, music and videotapes received by a child may have a biblical theme. A child's artwork made during hospitalization provides important hints about what the child is thinking.

The child's close relationships give information pertinent to spiritual assessment. For example, does the child have a parent or other significant adult present, or does she spend long periods alone? Are interactions with family members nurturing and supportive of the child? Does the child have visitors from church or Sunday school?

Asking the Right Questions

After these systematic observations are made, their meaning and significance to the child must be interpreted and validated. As observations are made, nurses can reflect on the child's behavior to ascertain the accuracy of their interpretations. For example, a nurse can say, "You seem sad [or angry, or afraid] today, Jonathan." A nurse can comment on environmental cues by saying, "I see you have a Bible. Do you have a favorite Bible story? What do you like about that story?"

Questions can be a natural response to daily events occurring during hospitalization. Spontaneous questions may be more effective in eliciting spiritual concerns than a thorough interview, because families may feel more comfortable sharing this information in a less structured situation. Potential areas of spiritual need will arise out of circumstances in our daily care of children.

Taking a faith history is the cornerstone to thorough spiritual assessment. A faith history unlocks the door to the meaning of behavioral, verbal and environmental observations. According to Ruth Stoll, the timing of the interview can either enhance or inhibit open sharing of information. The faith history can be incorporated into the admission nursing history. The rationale for asking spiritual questions is to enhance knowledge of sources of strength and should be shared with the families.[4]

Questions about the importance of faith in a healthcare crisis should not be limited solely to the admission history. These questions can be used at any time when the information may be helpful in providing supportive care to a child and family. As the nurse's relationship with each family is unique, so will be the degree of spiritual assessment that is appropriate for the situation. The nurse must be aware that the values or beliefs elicited by the questions may not be expressed through traditional religious language.[5]

A faith history should begin with questions for the parent. However, from the late preschool or early school period, children may be able to give important information about spiritual needs. Children should be given the opportunity to answer age-appropriate questions about their faith, faith practices and what or who helps them during difficult times. Some children will be able to give direct answers to questions. Younger and less verbally sophisticated children may give information through artwork, pictures, stories or play.

Stoll identified four areas of spiritual concern that should be covered in a spiritual assessment: concept of God, sources of hope and strength, religious practices, and thoughts about the relationship between beliefs and health.[6] The Spiritual Assessment list (see page 196) identifies potential questions that can be asked of parents and children during a spiritual assessment.

We have discussed the importance of understanding a child's development, along with the importance of accurate assessment and history-taking. Where do we go from here? Jesus said in Mark 10:14, ". . . Let the little children come to me; do not stop them; for it is to such as these that the kingdom of God belongs."

Use of Self to Meet Spiritual Needs

How do we intervene spiritually for children and their families? One way that nurses can care for children spiritually is through using ourselves. Judith Shelly and Sharon Fish describe key elements in the therapeutic use of self, including listening, empathy, vulnerability, humility and commitment.[7]

Spending time with pediatric patients provides us with an opportunity to listen effectively. Periods of listening may occur during the normal caregiving times. However, we may need to carve out quiet, uninterrupted time to focus on the child. A child might be thinking in a deeper way than they are able to express. Children need to be watched closely, while using good listening skills, to discern their thoughts and feelings. If what we are hearing from the child is not consistent with the child's behavior, the child may be letting us know his concern and distress.

A child's thinking may not be logical. She may truly believe that a ghost is under her bed or that when her parents leave, she will never see them again. The words we use and the expectations we have must be consistent with the child's stage of development. Children may express thoughts through play that they would not be able to communicate verbally.

Empathy is the ability to experience another's emotions or feelings. Nurses can become empathetic by trying to put themselves in the place of the child. Empathy is more than an intellectual response, sympathy or feeling sorry for a child. Empathy is the art of understanding a child's feelings and remaining objective enough to assist the child in whatever manner necessary. The world looks very different through the eyes of a child. Our ability to empathize will help children trust us and enable them to feel safe and secure.

Being vulnerable allows others to see who we really are. By becoming vulnerable, nurses are able to lend strength to patients and families. Becoming vulnerable can be very threatening. Many nurses are parents themselves. It is difficult to stand by a parent who watches a child suffer and struggle with illness. Nurses who are vulnerable risk being hurt, but they also allow themselves to minister to children and families in a deep, meaningful way.

Humility is an ability to recognize our limitations, something nurses often struggle with. When caring for pediatric patients, remember what Jesus said in Matthew 18:4, "Whoever becomes humble like this child is the greatest in the kingdom of heaven." Jesus holds the child up as an example for us and provides a perfect model to follow. Parents of hospitalized children are often confused and frightened. Modeling humility, the nurse not only functions as an expert but serves also as a helpful and available resource.

Making a commitment to patients means promising your presence for as long as they need support.[8] Nurses become willing to share in pain and suffering through the tough times as well as the good.

It takes a great deal of strength to use ourselves in this way. Ultimately, commitment is the reflection of God's relationship with humanity.[9] Through God's strength, the nurse who is committed offers patients an unending resource and support.

Use of Touch to Meet Spiritual Needs

Another way nurses can intervene spiritually with children is through touch. The biblical basis for the use of touch is found in Mark 10:13, "People were bringing little children to him in order that he might touch them . . . " Nurses must be aware of which parts of the body are most appropriate to touch. Stroking a child's hand or arm may remind him of your presence. Rocking a small child, braiding a girl's hair or rubbing a child's back may provide a concrete way for us to connect with and comfort children. Touch can be a wonderful way of soothing a child who has gone through a painful procedure or simply misses his parents.

John, a hospitalized eighteen-year-old, was dying of leukemia. John's family visited infrequently. The first day that John's nurse cared for him, she noticed how depressed and hopeless he seemed. During a quiet moment one afternoon, she asked John if he would like her to rub his back. John readily accepted and stated that she was the first person who had touched him since he had been in the hospital. John had been on the unit for one month and felt totally isolated from people. Through touch, the nurse reached out and comforted John.

Use of Prayer and Scripture to Meet Spiritual Needs

Prayer may also be used to provide spiritual care for children and families. Prayer may be described as a time of reflection and communication with God. Prayer may be a quieting, peaceful time focused on God as a source of strength and hope. Many times, however, during crisis and illness, individuals become distanced from God. Some may feel anger and bitterness, possibly even betrayal. Through prayer, nurses may be able to build a bridge between children and God.

Jennifer had been caring for a newborn with Down Syndrome and a life-threatening heart defect since his birth four hours previously. As she entered his mother's darkened room, she found Linda crying softly. Jennifer quietly approached her, put her hand on Linda's arm and spent the next few minutes sharing about Linda's son. Linda expressed her grief and fear over the possibility of his death.

At the end of their time together, Jennifer asked Linda if she would like her to pray for them. Linda nodded in agreement, and Jennifer prayed: "Dear God, please comfort Linda tonight. Keep Linda and her son safe, and help them to feel your presence. Amen."

As Jennifer cared for Linda and her son over the next few days, Linda introduced Jennifer to family and friends as "the nurse who prayed with me." Jennifer then realized what an important part of her nursing care this prayer had been.

When should we pray with children and their families? Children may enjoy mealtime or bedtime prayer. School-age children and adolescents can be asked directly if they would like to pray. Times of stress and anxiety may create a need in the child to reach out to God. The obvious times of fear, suffering and death seem particularly important. Three-year-old Kari prayed, "Dear Jesus, I have something important to tell you. Grandma died, and she is in heaven with you, Jesus, and I miss her." Kari felt closer to her grandmother by talking to Jesus.

We may pray for our patients as part of our personal prayer time, and we may let them know we are praying for them. Rolf Garborg, in his book *The Blessing*, talks about our ability to bestow a blessing upon individuals, an intentional act of speaking God's favor and power into someone's life.[10] Mark 10 describes how Jesus took the children in his arms and blessed them, laying his hands upon them. Offering a blessing to a child may remind her of God's love for her and his presence with her. A good blessing to use is found in Numbers 6:24-26, "The Lord bless you and keep you; the Lord make his face to shine upon you, and be gracious to you; the Lord lift up his countenance upon you, and give you peace."

The nurse may use conversational or shared prayer, as Jennifer did, when both the nurse and the patient feel comfortable and want to pray. The prayer itself can be short and simple. It can reflect the child's feelings, fears and concerns, opening the lines of communication between the child and God. After spiritual assessment, the nurse will be able to provide prayer for patients in a comfortable, appropriate and meaningful manner.

Sharing religious materials, Bible stories or Scripture verses with children may be helpful and offer an additional source of comfort. Once again, it is important to carefully assess children's desire for this intervention and select suitable stories or verses.

Melissa was preparing to send a four-year-old patient to surgery. After observing his mother reading the Bible, Melissa asked if she might share one of her favorite passages. Not only did the child's mother accept this offer, she also asked Melissa to pray with them, asking God for strength for the family, sustaining them through the long hours ahead. Melissa shared Scripture during a family's time of fear and apprehension.

We may read Bible stories, Scripture or devotional material to children when they are struggling to fall asleep or experiencing pain during illness. Children love stories and often learn deep spiritual truths from them. During periods of loneliness and moments of sadness, families may find comfort in hearing God's Word.

Choosing the appropriate Scripture passage is as important as the timing of when it is read. Verses giving comfort and strength are those that remind us of God's presence and hope. When relating to children, nurses need to share verses or stories that the child is able to understand.

Is Sharing Your Faith Appropriate?

Should nurses share their faith? Are we withholding a helpful intervention if we choose not to share our faith at appropriate times? No consensus among Christian nurses can be found in this area of spiritual care. But we believe that we can share our faith, based on a careful assessment and identification of the child's spiritual need, and not on a personal need or desire.

George Handzo offers some practical thoughts for nurses discussing faith issues with children. A nurse should answer questions children ask by giving brief answers and refraining from expounding on deep, abstract theological concepts. He also encourages nurses to avoid offending children or devaluing their beliefs.[11] God's love for children is something they can cling to during fearful times. We offer our faith experience as a way of providing hope, not as a way of undermining the child's existing belief system. By our accepting, respectful spirit, we give children an example of a person of faith. The child can see by our actions that our love is a reflection of God's love and care for them.

When ministering to children spiritually, it is important to remember all the resources available to us. The hospital chaplain and the child's pastor or spiritual advisor can offer additional spiritual support. Sadly, the chaplain and the nurse often do not work together. In the midst of busy days on hospital units, nurses may believe spiritual needs are the responsibility of the chaplain, while physical and emotional needs remain in the nurse's realm of care.

The team effort of the nurse and the chaplain, however, can be extremely effective. Nurses spend a great deal of time with the children and families and, therefore, may know their needs and concerns. The nurse may need to refer difficult questions to the chaplain and may also request a spiritual leader's services for baptism, sacraments and other religious rituals. The chaplain also may become a safe, *uninvolved* individual in whom the child can comfortably confide.[12]

Looking back over your career, what times have given you the most meaning? The following letter was written to a nurse from a family whose newborn son died shortly before birth.

"Dear Ellen: I don't know that Jim and I can ever thank you for all you've done for us these past days. Thank you for being there when we discovered our baby had died, for encircling me with your arms and weeping with me at the unfairness of it all. Thank you for not leaving us alone in our grief. For placing little Johnny in our arms, for saying hello with us and for saying goodbye. For visiting with us, for touching my leg and holding Jim's hand. For encouraging Jim and me to have a memorial service for Johnny, so that others might remember him with us."

Ellen demonstrated God's love to this family through the use of empathy, vulnerability, commitment and touch. The spiritual care she delivered had a tremendous impact and enabled the parents to begin grieving the loss of their son. The systematic use of the nursing process provides nurses with the framework to assess our patients and use spiritual interventions. As nurses, we can respond to children and families as Ellen did, making a significant difference in people's lives.

Originally published in JCN, Spring, 1995

NOTES

1 Judith A. Shelly, *The Spiritual Needs of Children* (Downers Grove, Ill.: InterVarsity Press, 1982), p. 81.

2 Judith V. Still, "How to Assess Spiritual Needs of Children and Their Families," *Journal of Christian Nursing* 1, no. 1 (1984): 5.

3 Verna B. Carson, *Spiritual Dimensions of Nursing Practice* (Philadelphia: W. B. Saunders, 1989), p. 158.

4 Ruth Stoll, "Guidelines for Spiritual Assessment," *American Journal of Nursing* 79, no. 9 (1979): 1577.

5 Ibid.

[6] Ibid., 1574.

[7] Judith A. Shelly & Sharon Fish, *Spiritual Care: The Nurse's Role,* 3rd edition (Downers Grove, Ill.: InterVarsity Press, 1988), pp. 96, 98, 101, 103.

[8] Carson, *Spiritual Dimensions,* p. 168.

[9] Shelly & Fish, *Spiritual Care,* p. 104.

[10] Rolf Garborg, *The Family Blessing* (Dallas: Word, 1990), p. 13.

[11] George Handzo, "Talking About Faith with Children," *Journal of Christian Nursing* 7, no. 4 (1990): 20.

[12] Carson, *Spiritual Dimensions,* p. 173.

26

Ages & Stages of Spiritual Development

Sue Steen & Betsy Anderson

When Shannon's first-grade friend, Katie, was hospitalized with a brain tumor, she questioned her mom and dad. "Why did Katie get sick? Is God going to let her die?"

At an early age, children experience a variety of losses, illnesses and accidents in their everyday lives. They need help in understanding the meaning of these experiences and placing them in perspective.

Pediatric nurses have been given the challenging responsibility of providing care for children and families. Children's spiritual needs are closely related to their physical, psychosocial and developmental needs. Many nurses provide excellent physical and emotional care but overlook the deeper spiritual needs precipitated by illness. Spiritual care of children should be incorporated into the total plan of care for the child and family.

In our national climate of respect for diversity, it may be difficult as Christian nurses to know how to incorporate the spiritual care of children and families into our practice. Children of diverse backgrounds need to be viewed as special gifts of God, regardless of differences in belief systems. All people must be treated with respect, even if we disagree with their beliefs.

Who is better positioned to assess and meet the spiritual needs of children and families than the nurse who is caring for them? To do so, we must ask several questions: What do children believe? What are a child's spiritual needs? How do we identify these needs and give spiritual care to children and families?

What Do Children Believe About God?

Amy was three when she asked her mother to sing "Turn Your Eyes upon Jesus" at bedtime. As her mother was singing, Amy kept lifting up her head and looking around the room. Her mother said, "Amy, lay your head down and go to sleep."

"No, Mom," Amy said. "I'm turning my eyes to Jesus."

Stories like these show us that during the early years, children are thinking about faith issues. George Handzo says we should not confuse children's inability to talk about God with an inability to think about or appreciate God.[1] Children think differently from adults. They often may be unable to express their faith concerns, thus creating a need for our understanding of faith development in children.

The nursing literature reflects different opinions on how children develop spiritually. Many researchers, however, found that spiritual development occurs in stages.

Authors J. Roland Fleck, Stanley Ballard and J. Wesley Reilly describe data from many different researchers studying religious development in children. They found that religious deveopment consistently correlates with Piaget's stages of cognitive development. They delineated religious developmental stages that corresponded closely with Jean Piaget's preoperational, concrete operational and formal operational periods.[2]

Ernest Harms described how children think about and conceptualize God. He asked children to draw pictures of how God would look. The results showed three broad classes of drawings reflecting different themes of a child's understanding of God.

Three- to six-year-old children drew God as a king living in the clouds. Seven- to twelve-year-olds began to separate their personal fantasy from reality and viewed God in terms of faith symbols such as crucifixes and Jewish stars. Thirteen- to eighteen-year-olds viewed God in different ways. One group maintained a conventional view of God, while others viewed God abstractly through sunrises and rainbows.[3]

Diane Long studied children's understanding of prayer and again found three major developmental stages. Children moved from a vague, indistinct understanding of prayer to a stage where they viewed prayer as a routine, external activity, rather than personal communication with God. During the third stage, children viewed prayer as a private conversation with God. At this stage, their prayers are less egocentric and more altruistic.[4]

James Fowler, whose work was influenced by Piaget, formulated a six-stage model of children's cognitive faith development. He defined faith as the knowing by which persons recognize themselves as related to the transcendent, or God. Children initially base their faith on egocentrism and fantasy, while imitating religious behavior of parents. God is understood in magical terms. Later they begin to separate religious understanding from fantasy and have a concrete, literal interpretation of faith symbols. For example, children view heaven as in the sky, and the cross as a wooden structure upon which Jesus died. During this stage, if children have a relationship with God, they base it on what God can give them.

During the next stage, Fowler found that children begin to look to authority to reconcile conflicting beliefs, and then begin to internalize their individual belief in God. At this stage, they are greatly influenced by others and the values of their group of friends. Individuals may continue to develop spiritually throughout their lifetime or may stay at an earlier stage of spiritual development.[5]

Erik Erikson's theory of psychosocial development is the foundation for LeRoy Aden's work on eight stages of faith. Aden looks at faith as a developmental phenomenon, determined in part by the stage in which the individual is engaged. The infant begins faith development with a sense of trust. The child then moves through stages of courage during the toddler years, while developing faith through obedience during the preschool years.

As the child begins school, he enters the assent stage of faith and "wholeheartedly accepts God." During the last stage of childhood, the adolescent develops faith as it relates to his identity.[6]

Not everyone agrees that religious or spiritual development occurs in stages; further research is needed in this area. However, there are advantages for nurses who use the stage theory in understanding a child's faith development.

Most nurses are familiar with Piaget's and Erikson's theories of cognitive and psychosocial development and so can apply their understanding of these theories to the spiritual realm of their patients. Nurses can then better understand the child's spiritual thoughts, beliefs and concerns.

Dear God,
Thank you for the baby brother but what I prayed for was a puppy
Joyce

The stage theory may not apply to every child in all situations. We know that children vary developmentally, and this must be remembered when working with them. The stage theory, however, gives us a place to begin spiritual care.

How Do Spiritual Needs Relate to Stages?

Though children's spiritual needs may be similar to adults', they are expressed differently, based on the child's development. Children have a need for love and relationship, a need for forgiveness and a need for meaning, purpose and hope in life.[7]

Dear Mr. God

I wish you would not make it so easy for people to come apart. I had 3 stitches and a shot.

Janet

Infants: Infants are known by God and have a spiritual dimension similar to people of all ages. The earliest spiritual need to appear is the need for unconditional love.[8] An infant first experiences this unconditional love in early relationships with a parent. As infants grow and develop, the relationship with parents provides a foundation for trust in God. Children develop a sense of trust, belonging and self-worth as they learn that their needs will be consistently met by the parent. This provides the prerequisite for development of a relationship with God, as the child grows in understanding.

The dependence of a baby on her mother reflects the relationship between the Creator and those created. The individual approaches God with the same openness and receptivity that characterizes the infant's approach to a mother.[9]

As infants are loved, cuddled, comforted, talked to and protected from harm, they are able to grow to be physically, emotionally and spiritually healthy.

Under normal circumstances these needs can be met quite easily. However, they are not met as easily when a child is in a hospital setting. Many hospitalized children are routinely poked and prodded. They have their feeding and sleep schedules interrupted and experience many new sounds and faces, all of which create a frightening impression.

Parents need permission to provide a safe, comfortable environment for their child during hospitalization. They can be encouraged to try and keep their child on a normal daily schedule. As nurses, we can advocate for our clients by encouraging other members of the health care team to honor the child's needs whenever that is possible.

Nurses may also find themselves filling in for unavailable parents and becoming the child's consistent caretaker for days, weeks or months. Matthew was two days old when diagnosed with a meconium ileus related to cystic fibrosis. His mother had no choice but to return to her rural home one hundred miles away to care for her four other children. During his two-week hospitalization, Sue consistently cared for Matthew and talked with his mother every day. His mother valued the nursing care Matthew was receiving. Sixteen years later, Sue still receives an annual Christmas card and picture of Matthew. She believes God allowed her to play a part in Matthew's emotional and spiritual development.

Toddlers: According to Erikson, the toddler's quest is to become autonomous. Through the process of separation from parents, becoming somewhat independent and asserting their wills, toddlers begin to feel a sense of self worth.[10] Author Verna Carson states that children must have a healthy self-worth to become intimate with God. Children's ability to love themselves leads to their ability to feel love from God.[11]

Even in the hospital, toddlers must know what is expected of them. Clear expectations create a more predictable environment for toddlers, allowing them to meet with success rather than failure. Consistent caregivers, along with predictability in the daily schedule, will provide toddlers with a sense of security in knowing what to anticipate each day. The toddler may also enjoy religious rituals, such as prayer before meals and bedtime. Parents may tell us which prayers the child can recite, as well as favorite bedtime stories.

Preschoolers: Preschoolers are learning about the world through their experiences. They begin to balance self-assertion and self-discipline. They are learning to control their desires, while meeting expectations of others. As they work on self-discipline, they simultaneously need to feel unconditional love. Unrealistic demands may cause them to continually feel inadequate. During this stage, children begin to develop a conscience that tells them about right and wrong.[12] When children feel guilty or bad about themselves, their feelings affect their relationships. They may view themselves as unacceptable or inadequate to be loved by others or by God.

Four-year-old Jason slept very little the night of his hospital admission. The nurse brought in his breakfast tray and set it on the bedside table in front of him. Before anyone realized what was happening, Jason pushed the tray of food off his table and onto the floor.

Many of us have had a similar experience. Our initial reaction is often one of anger, frustration and feelings of futility. It is tempting to respond angrily, walk away or ignore Jason. What would help Jason and keep this from happening again? Jason must know our expectations of him but also must know we will not turn our back on him. Nurses can provide unconditional love for the child by being available. Children must feel accepted, regardless of their behavior. By our continual presence and care for preschoolers, we provide them with security.

This can be difficult. We may not feel like responding in this manner, and it may not be something we can do every day. However, this is a patient-care approach we can strive for and ask God to help us provide.

School-age children: School-age children are learning and growing through producing and accomplishing things.[13] Through their mastery of knowledge and skills, children begin to feel competent and successful. School-age children may spend time thinking about what God does and how he does it. They may still combine concrete, logical thought with fantasy. Often, to enhance their spiritual understanding, school-age children ask detailed questions about how God works.

School-age children believe in good and evil, which may lead to feelings of fear and guilt. Because of these feelings, the child has the spiritual need for forgiveness and freedom from guilt. Based on their cognitive development, school-age children may believe that illness, hospitalizations or death are punishments for their wrong thoughts or behavior. At this stage, children need to know that God does not punish children for misdeeds by making them sick or by making tragic events happen.

Children at this age need to concretely experience forgiveness in their human relationships, as well as in their relationship with God. They need to know that God has not abandoned them, and that God offers forgiveness. Children often need help in resolving guilt feelings about their role in illness, accidents or death. They also may need help in dealing with angry feelings at God. Nurses can be attentive to what children are thinking about their circumstances and listen as they struggle to understand difficult events. Frequently, a child's misconceptions can be corrected, lifting the burden of guilt. A child also can learn of the forgiveness Jesus offers when we confess our wrongdoing and trust in the power of his death to restore the relationship with our loving God.

Adolescents: Adolescents are striving for individuality and identity. They desire to become independent from their parents and determine who they are and what they believe.[14] They are capable of developing a deep relationship with God. The spiritual need that arises in adolescence is the need for meaning, purpose and hope in life.[15] This spiritual need requires the development of abstract-thought processes, often seen in Piaget's stage of formal operations.

The search for purpose and meaning in life corresponds with Erikson's stage of identity versus role confusion. Beginning in the adolescent years, people need to make sense out of life, as well as find some meaning in suffering and illness. In the midst of difficulties, adolescents need hope that God is in control, is present and can support them through difficult times.

Emily had been hospitalized numerous times with Crohn's disease. Each time she was admitted, she became more and more despondent. Her depression led her to withdraw from staff and become noncompliant with treatment. Emily was struggling with many difficult questions: Why was she allowed to suffer? Was she ever going to get well?

Emily did not need to hear about God's plan in her suffering, but she did need to know that nurses would be present to listen and support her. She needed to feel care and concern in human relationships as a reflection of God's care and love for her. The nurses who cared for Emily became faithful models of Christ as she worked through painful issues.

Handzo says that what children need and want spiritually is to be loved and cared for by a benevolent and forgiving God. They need to know that despite anything they think or do, God forgives and never leaves them. Most of all, they need the hope that comes from knowing God has not abandoned them.[16] These themes can be recognized in interactions with children of different developmental levels.

Four-year-old Amy's prayer before Sunday dinner reflects these developmental themes and spiritual needs. She prayed, "Dear Jesus, please come down to earth so we can see you real soon. Don't ever die again. And keep away all the bad guys." Amy's simple prayer demonstrates her concrete concept of God and elementary understanding of death, as well as her need for the protecting presence of a loving God. Nurses who are aware of children's spiritual development can recognize their understanding of God and spiritual concerns, and can use this to plan developmentally appropriate spiritual care for children and their families.

Originally published in JCN, *Spring, 1995*

NOTES

[1] George Handzo, "Talking About Faith with Children," *Journal of Christian Nursing* 7, no. 4 (1990): 18.

[2] J. Roland Fleck, Stanley N. Ballard & J. Wesley Reilly, "The Development of Religious Concepts and Maturity: a Three-Stage Model," *Journal of Psychology and Theology* 3, no. 3 (1975): 156.

[3] Ernest Harms, "The Development of Religious Experience in Children," *American Journal of Sociology* 50 (1944): 112-22.

[4] Diane Long, David Elkind & Bernard Spilka, "The Child's Conception of Prayer," *Journal for the Scientific Study of Religion* 6, no. 1 (1967): 101.

[5] James Fowler, "Toward a Developmental Perspective on Faith," *Religious Education* 69, no. 2 (1974): 214-17.

[6] LeRoy Aden, "Faith and the Developmental Cycle," *Pastoral Psychology* 24, no. 3 (1976): 217.

[7] Judith A. Shelly & Sharon Fish, *Spiritual Care: The Nurse's Role*, 3rd edition (Downers Grove, Ill.: InterVarsity Press, 1988), p. 40.

[8] Judith V. Still, "Assessing Spiritual Needs of Children and Their Families," in Judith A. Shelly, *The Spiritual Needs of Children* (Downers Grove, Ill.: InterVarsity Press, 1982), p. 93.

[9] Verna B. Carson, *Spiritual Dimensions of Nursing Practice* (Philadelphia: W. B. Saunders, 1989), p. 35.

[10] Erik Erikson, *Childhood and Society* (New York: Norton, 1963), p. 252.

[11] Carson, *Spiritual Dimensions*, p. 35.

[12] Erikson, *Childhood and Society*, p. 256.

[13] Ibid., p. 259.

[14] Ibid., p. 261.

[15] Shelly, *The Spiritual Needs of Children*, p. 96.

[16] Handzo, "Talking About Faith," p. 18.

27

Congregational Care
Reaching Out to the Elderly

Mary Ellen Lashley

What a glorious Sunday morning! Sunbeams sparkled brightly as the organ played familiar hymns. The people filed into the rapidly filling sanctuary, greeting friends and finding their favorite seats. Feeling content, I settled into my pew, ready to worship. Then, suddenly, a deacon approached me, looking apprehensive. "Clara's not feeling well. She's sitting in the back of the church, complaining of chest pain. I picked her up at home in the church van this morning. She said she ran out of her medicine. I asked her if she wanted to stay home or call the doctor, but she says that if she's going to die, she wants to die in the church, where she will be surrounded by her friends."

Clara, eighty-two years old, had a history of unstable angina. I knew her well, having visited her home on many occasions. As the parish nurse for this small Baptist congregation, I cared for many of our elderly members.

I went to the back of the church where Clara sat. It was evident after chatting with her briefly that her chest pain was of cardiac origin. However, she refused to go to the hospital. Assessing her medications, I discovered she had run out of nitroglycerin. I informed the pastor and church leaders of this medically unstable member in the service. The choir director remarked, "The organist takes nitroglycerin for angina. I wonder if it's the same thing."

Immediately, I located the organist to ask if she had some nitroglycerin with her. Securing a tablet, I then broke a cardinal rule of medication administration: never share a medicine prescribed for you with another person.

One nitroglycerin did the trick. Clara experienced relief of her pain within minutes. After assessing that she was stable, I secured the number of her doctor and called to inform him of the episode and her need for a prescription renewal. He called the pharmacy, and I picked up her medicine, delivering it to her just in time to hear the end of the sermon. Such was one Sunday morning in my life as a parish nurse.

Parish nursing is a relatively new professional nursing role that has drawn much interest from the nursing community in recent years. Yet, in many ways, it is simply a return to the original mission of the church: ministering to the sick and infirm in the community. Historically, the clergy and the religious orders provided care for the sick and disenfranchised in society. Parish nursing, then, is a missionary outreach to the community.[1]

The parish nurse role is challenging, full of opportunities for innovative care delivery. The concept of congregation-based health care is particularly relevant to the elderly. Between one-third and one-fourth of the members of most faith communities are over sixty-five.[2] Most members are older persons who embrace and affirm spiritual values. The parish nurse can meet the health care needs of the elderly, enhance their self-esteem, address their spiritual needs and assist them to meet the developmental tasks of older adulthood.

The congregational care model for delivery of health services was renewed in the 1980s by Granger Westberg, a Lutheran minister and hospital chaplain.[3] He saw the role of the nurse as pivotal in addressing the health care needs of the faith community. The parish nurse is a member of the ministry team, who provides holistic care to members of the congregation.[4]

There has been little standardization in terms of requirements or scope of practice for parish nurses, but this is changing. Nurses with varied levels of education and experience may work on either a paid or volunteer basis to address the health care needs of a congregation. However, it is the registered, baccalaureate or higher degree prepared nurse who has the broad background in community health, leadership and research to more fully meet the physical, emotional and spiritual needs of the older adult.

The parish nurse is in a unique role to address the spiritual needs of the older client. By delivering care in the client's home or place of worship, the nurse is in an environment that is personally meaningful to the older client.[5] The relationship, then, becomes more egalitarian and less hierarchical. Clients retain control and maintain a sense of comfort in knowing their source of care comes from their faith community.

The parish nurse has a unique opportunity to see the client in meaningful interactions with others and in worship. The client's spiritual beliefs and values are recognized and respected, and conversations about spirituality flow naturally. The client is encouraged to explore the meaning of prayer, suffering and belief in God to build strength and to cope with adversity.[6] The client is fully supported in his or her faith.

A meaningful program to address clients' physical, emotional and spiritual needs in our church has been a "Super Seniors" group led by a special lady, a highly gifted woman in the church with a background in recreational and music therapy. After submitting a survey to the seniors in the church to find out what activities would be most meaningful to them, the seniors' group was formed. The group is wellness-focused and meets monthly. A typical meeting includes a time of prayer, devotions and group activities that include physical exercise, memory enhancing exercises and therapeutic reminiscence. Reminiscence allows older persons to find meaning in the significant past events that have shaped their lives, to come to terms with unresolved conflicts and to deal with past losses.[7]

Guest speakers present a variety of health promotion topics including nutrition, fitness, medication management and elder law. Through this group, our seniors have developed meaningful social interactions. Outcomes include a decrease in depressive symptomatology, improved affect, greater involvement in social activities and reports of an increased sense of meaning and purpose. Group-sponsored senior day-trips are by far the most popular activities.

A home visitation ministry is another powerful tool for meeting the health care needs in our congregation. Nurses and deacons make visits, at times jointly, to members who are sick and homebound. Nursing services provided in the home include blood pressure screening and physical assessment, medication assessment and teaching, fall prevention and home safety education, therapeutic reminiscence and referral and resource coordination.

Many of our homebound elderly are fragile, potentially unstable and at risk for institutionalization. These services help clients to maintain their independence and prevent injury and premature hospitalization. In addition, both client and family members are comforted to know that chronic medical conditions are monitored on a regular basis in the convenience of the client's home without cost to the client. In addition, the clients feel they are not forgotten by the church and appreciate the opportunity to socialize and fellowship with others in the faith community.

A wonderful addition to our nursing ministry has been the involvement of student nurses from a local university. Since I teach community health nursing, I can bring nursing students into the church to learn health promotion and public health principles. The students visit our elders at home, attend services with their clients and participate in the wellness ministries of the church (blood pressure screening clinics, health teaching to different age groups in the Sunday school, participation in the Super Seniors group).

Student nurse involvement has become a powerful and highly effective ministry for our older clients and a valuable learning experience for the students. For clients, this experience provides an opportunity to develop a grandparenting relationship with our students. The older clients feel they are sharing their wisdom and nurturing the next generation of young people and, in so doing, meet a vital developmental task of older adulthood. On the other hand, the students learn how personal faith can sustain persons through the many crises they encounter in their lives. They see their clients in an environment that defines them and is meaningful to them. They begin to grasp that there is more to growing older than suffering from a chronic illness.

Moreover, the students are challenged to view their work as more than a profession, as a calling: a call to care for those in need and to minister to persons wherever they may be found. Students are challenged to question the existing boundaries of their practice and to recognize innovative and creative ways to reach elders with unmet health care needs.

My faculty colleagues sometimes express concern about how students of different faith perspectives, or no organized faith, can feel comfortable providing nursing care in an environment that is strongly Christ-centered. How can students practice without feeling proselytized or pressured to conform?

Interestingly, in the three years I have had students in this setting, they have never voiced this concern. Although students attend services with their clients and hear their personal stories, they report feeling more secure, accepted and free to be themselves than in any other nursing practice setting. The church, then, nurtures the authenticity of the nurse, as well as the client. Students hear the gospel message from the testimonies of their clients who have suffered multiple losses and have found their faith in Christ to be their strength. Some students have reported that they grew up in a place of worship but strayed from it as young adults. Their experiences in the parish nurse rotation have actually brought them back to their childhood faith and helped them to regain the spiritual side of themselves, which they thought they had lost.

The parish nurse role is a unique, nontraditional one that poses great opportunities for meeting the needs of older persons in the community. Through an interdisciplinary, congregational care model, the nurse collaborates with medical professionals and church leaders to plan holistic care to promote physical, emotional and spiritual well-being. In an era of managed health care delivery and shortened hospital stays, nurses need to consider finding new places for ministering to the older client that are innovative and community-based. The parish nurse role allows the nurse to be present to older clients within their places of worship and to draw on their spiritual resources to find hope and strength to cope in times of adversity.

Originally published in JCN, *Summer, 1999*

NOTES

[1] Maria T. Boario, "Mercy Model: Church-Based Health Care in the Inner City," *Journal of Christian Nursing* 10, no. 1 (Winter 1993): 20-22 **(in Chap. 16, pg. 125 of this publication)**; Ann Solari-Twadell and Granger Westberg, "Body, Mind and Soul: The Parish Nurse Offers Physical, Emotional and Spiritual Care," *Health Progress* (September 1991): 24-28.

[2] Twadell and Westberg: 24-28.

[3] Granger Westberg, "Parish Nurses: Specialists in Wellness Care," *The Christian Ministry* (November-December 1991): 9-11.

[4] Mary Jane Schank, Darlene Weis and Rose Marie Matheus, "Parish Nursing: Ministry of Healing," *Geriatric Nursing* 17, no. 1 (1996): 11-13.

[5] Mary Lashley, "Reminiscence: A Biblical Basis for Telling Our Stories," *Journal of Christian Nursing* 9, no. 3 (Summer 1992): 4-8.

[6] Marsha Davis, "The Rehabilitation Nurse's Role in Spiritual Care," *Rehabilitation Nursing* 19, no. 5 (1994): 298-301.

[7] Mary Lashley, "The Painful Side of Reminiscence," *Geriatric Nursing* 14, no. 3 (1993): 138-41.

Part Six

Issues in Congregational Health

28

Nursing Ethics
Growing Beyond Rules of Conduct

Susan A. Salladay

As a dedicated breeder of purebred Standard Poodles and Salukis, I know that the judges who evaluate my dogs in the show ring look for breed *type*. "Type" is hard to define but is always in reference to a specific category (in the case of purebred dogs, it's the breed standard as defined by the parent club for the breed). One author puts it this way: "[Type is] the elusive quality that makes [a dog] *look like* the breed."[1] Type is essence.

As a nurse-ethicist, I want to explore the *type*, the essence, of ethics (behaviors, responsibilities and values) most characteristic of the profession of nursing. Ethical theories are many and varied. Is nursing marked by an elusive quality in its professional ethics and values that makes it look like what it is? In other words, are nurses distinguished by what they do morally?

And is what they do essentially Christian? Are the moral values embodied in nursing distinctively Christian?

Nursing's origins and its identity, ethics and values are complex and multifaceted. According to M. Patricia Donahue, "From the dawn of civilization, evidence prevails to support the premise that *nurturing* has been essential to the preservation of life. Survival of the human race, therefore, is inextricably intertwined with the development of nursing. . . . Nursing has been called the oldest of the arts and the youngest of the professions."[2]

Donahue considers the origins of nursing through the etymology of the words *nurse* and *to nurse,* noting that the word *nursing* is derived from the Latin *nutrire* (to nourish) and *nutrix* (nursing mother). The noun *nurse* was derived from the 13th-century English word *nurice,* which meant "wet nurse" (a woman who suckled a child not her own) and, by the 16th century, included the meaning "a person who waits upon or tends the sick."[3]

Donahue asserts that nursing is as old as medicine "although some . . . believe that nursing began with Florence Nightingale." She claims that the maternal instinct "provided the strong impulse or motive necessary to care for those who were suffering or helpless. As nursing care became more complex, it became apparent that factors other than a strong motive were necessary to do the work of a nurse. Yet this motivation continued to be a vital component of nursing's development. . . . It produced altruism or humanitarianism, the noblest form of love and kindness. Compelling societal forces such as religious fervor reinforced this motive . . . [but] love and caring alone were not sufficient to nurture health or overcome disease. The development of nursing depended on. . . skill. . . expertness and knowledge. . . The head, the hands and the heart became truly united to provide the strong foundation for modern-day nursing. The neglect . . . of any of these would provide for an imbalance in care."[4]

Donahue observes that from the earliest point in its history, the Christian church assumed a responsibility for the care of the sick. She notes that while other religions viewed suffering as deserved, therefore something to be left alone, "Christ specialized in relieving it. Christ's teachings of love and brotherhood transformed not only society but also the development of nursing. 'Organized nursing' was a direct response to these teachings and epitomized the concept of pure altruism."[5]

Biblical values are central to nursing ethics, significantly shaping its professional growth. They are the basis for ethical behavior, but Christianity is about more than doing good. It is essentially a faith of salvation; it's about what God did and does for us through Jesus Christ, more than what we are able to do for God. In Christianity our focus is always on Jesus, not ourselves (except in relation to him), and ethics and values must always be understood in context as the response of disciples to one who has rightfully claimed their allegiance as Lord and given them new life.

But priorities other than this have played a role in shaping nursing ethics. Gerald Winslow highlights the military metaphor "nursing as military effort in the battle against disease" that permeates many of the early discussions of nursing ethics: "[The military type] is associated with virtues such as loyalty and norms such as obedience to those of 'higher rank' and the maintenance of confidence in authority figures. . . Not only was modern nursing born in a military setting, it also emerged at a time when medicine was appropriating the military metaphor: medicine as war . . . disease is the *enemy* which threatens to *invade* the body and overwhelm its *defenses*. Medicine *combats* disease with *batteries* of tests and *arsenals* of drugs. . . . The goal of military discipline was to produce nurses with . . . the qualities of good soldiers.[6]

First attempts at delineating and expressing a distinctive code of ethics for nursing often combined medical-military imagery and values with those central to the Bible. Isabel Hampton Robb, principal of the Training School for Nurses at

Johns Hopkins Hospital, published one of the first textbooks about nursing ethics in 1900. She used military terminology in describing, for example, the correct conduct of the probationer (an individual not yet admitted to a training program but working on a ward under the supervision of a trained nurse who assessed her aptitude for nursing during the probationary period).

"Implicit, unquestioning obedience is one of the first lessons a probationer must learn. . . . The term of probation is calculated to discipline the beginner . . . for the work she will be expected to do . . . until she reaches a certain stage of thoroughness . . . and learns that each thing must be done not just any way, but that there is a right way. . . . The probationer will find that a certain military precision exists in regard to the deportment of a junior to those who are her superiors in office."[7]

In contrast to the issues-oriented focus addressed in nursing ethics today, early nursing ethics focused more on virtue ethics, describing the character and deportment of the ideal nurse. Robb distinguishes nursing ethics from etiquette: "By *ethics* is meant the science that treats human actions from a standpoint of right and wrong. It teaches men the practice of the duties of human life and the reasons for what they should do. . . . The rules of conduct adapted to the many diverse circumstances attending the nursing of the sick constitute *nursing ethics*. In addition to ethics, we employ another term. . . . *Etiquette*, speaking broadly, means a form of behavior or manners expressly or tacitly required on particular occasions. It makes up the code of polite life."[8]

Much of Robb's work on nursing ethics addresses what would now be characterized as nurses' demeanor or deportment. "Thus it is considered only courteous to stand when receiving an order or being spoken to by the superintendent, the head nurse or a physician."[9] Today this concern would hardly be an issue in nursing ethics. In fact, it would be subject to ridicule by some. Nursing ethics today is "issue oriented" (looking at types of moral problems) but is experiencing a renewed interest in "virtue ethics" (looking at the character of the good nurse). Careful reading shows Robb is working systematically to address the ethical significance of what we would now define as outcomes-oriented patient care.

"It is all-important to gain the goodwill and confidence of her patients and, in this connection, manners stand for much. To be companionable, a nurse must have a bright disposition, a serene, quiet cheerfulness, coupled with gentleness and decision of manner. Loudness and noise should be avoided; a harsh and abrupt or a hurried, fussy, excited manner grates upon the nerves. One should study to be quiet, deft and quick. Sick people are generally very easily disturbed by noise, and the sense of hearing is sometimes abnormally acute in illness, so that even ordinary sounds may cause positive suffering."[10]

In addressing what constitutes the "good nurse," Robb considers (as we do today) the concept of *professionalism* significant to nursing ethics. "But nurses are still reaching out toward ideals, which we trust may be realized in the fullness of time. In speaking of nursing as a *profession*, I use the term advisedly. Some prefer the term *vocation*, or the Anglo-Saxon word calling . . . the significance of a direct call from God to a consecrated service . . . and surely *profession* means all that *vocation* does and more . . . more responsibility, more serious duty, a higher skill and an employment needing an education more than that required in some other vocations of life."[11]

As nursing's culture and context became increasingly secular, the notion of vocation had already begun to assume second place, a lesser value in relation to that of a profession, losing its meaning and motivating power as a specific call from God, a divine impetus shaping an individual's future. Today in our educational system, for example, vocational training holds a lesser status than professional education.

Writing at the turn of the century, Robb clearly portrays Christian values as central to nursing ethics. In discussing what we today call *patient rights*, Robb counsels: "Let her resolve that her patients shall receive their due, or even more than their due, at her hands. . . . If she could only remember to follow in every [case] the golden rule . . . her ministrations would more nearly resemble those of him who pleased not himself but who came among men as a servant. The nearer to her heart she keeps the teachings and life of Christ in her everyday work, the greater will be her strength to overcome difficulties and to forget herself in helping others."[12]

Although Robb is generally more concerned with the character of the good nurse in developing a nursing ethic, she does consider several of the specific ethical dilemmas that nurses still find troublesome. For example, what should a nurse do if her responsibility to a patient conflicts with her obligation to uphold the physician-patient relationship? Robb prioritizes harmony over truth-telling. Notice her outcomes-oriented context.

"If [the nurse] is questioned by relatives, and she is really convinced in her own mind that . . . the patient is not getting the right treatment, it is not for her to give her judgment of the matter. It is far better to tell the inquirers . . . to confer with the attending physician and, if necessary, . . . to seek additional medical advice. . . . Cordial relations cannot fail to be established between physician and nurse when the latter proves herself to be his faithful and loyal assistant and he, in his turn, shows confidence in and respect for the nurse. . . . In brief, harmony in the sickroom is indispensable, if the best results are to be obtained."[13]

Decades after Robb, M. Josephine Flaherty also speaks of nursing's struggle for identity as a profession. "The 1980s are witnessing the overt striving of many . . . oppressed individuals and groups to attain recognition and status. Nursing, representing a significant group in society, is part of this movement as it seeks to establish itself as an identifiable profession that makes important contributions to the promotion of health and to the cure of illness. . . . The nursing profession is attempting to identify and to clarify nursing's unique role in society."[14]

However, Flaherty cites "the religious image" as one of three images acquired from history that "have tended to inhibit [nursing's] progress toward self-determined professionalism. The first . . . is the folk image of the nurse as mother. . . . Nursing skills were seen as experientially derived. . . . It was believed that nursing was not based on a body of knowledge and that no critical thought was required. . . . The second . . . from medieval times, is the religious image of the nurse as care-giver for the sick, who fulfilled her function as a Christian duty and a means to salvation. . . . This was . . . a vocation rather than a profession worthy of significant economic rewards. . . . The third image of the nurse as servant . . . emerged between the 16th and 19th centuries with the development of the Protestant-capitalistic ethic. . . . Nursing entered its 'Dark Ages' as ignorant and ill-paid women who accepted work as nurses as a last resort."[15]

It is interesting to note that Flaherty assumes that nurses saw in Christianity salvation that must be earned through doing one's "Christian duty" rather than received as a free gift from God to those who accept Jesus Christ as their Savior (Eph 2:8-9) and, therefore, understand medieval nursing as a duty or function believed to have provided a means of salvation. Flaherty also concedes that nursing would be better off seeing itself as a profession rather than a vocation that implies a duty of charity.

As nursing's culture and context become increasingly secular, biblical values function less as a foundation or typology for the development of nursing ethics. For example, in 1922 Dr. William H. Kilpatrick addressed the Department of Nursing and Health at the Teachers College alumni conference: "New and old elements are almost certain in a transition period like this to come into conflict. . . . Three factors . . . unite to produce the modern world . . . the growth and spread of science (or tested thought), the industrial revolution and the rise of democracy. . . . The external authority of Aristotle or of the church or of the Bible has yielded to the internal authority of inherent reason. . . . The external basis of authoritarian ethics is losing force."[16]

Because he saw traditional moral authorities having less influence, Kilpatrick called for the recognition of nursing as a self-governing profession with a code of professional ethics.

Although initial interest in a nursing code of ethics dates to the turn of the century,[17] it wasn't until 1926 that the American Nurses' Association first reviewed (but did not adopt) an ethical code. That first code of ethics described nursing as "an emerging profession" and urged nurses to practice the Golden Rule as "it embodies all that could be written in many pages on the relation of nurse to nurse."[18] In her history of the Code of Ethics for Nurses, Diane Viens notes that in 1935, the ANA's Committee on Ethical Standards began a study of professional codes and dilemmas nurses faced in practice.

In 1940 the committee presented a "tentative code" which, after revisions, was adopted in 1950 and revised in 1960, 1968 (the interpretive statements were added), 1976 (all gender references were deleted) and 1985. Reference to the Golden Rule was nowhere present in any later code.[19]

The development of nursing and nursing ethics is also intertwined with the development of hospitals and the practice of hospitalization of the sick. Anne Davis and Mila Aroskar observe that "the establishment of the first hospital occurred in India before the birth of Christ. As long as the sick remained at home, their care naturally fell to their families.

"With the shift from the home to the hospital, the services of some attendants to care for the sick, in addition to physicians, became a necessity. . . . Not until the Middle Ages did [hospitals] develop in Europe. . . . Our knowledge of nursing generally goes back to the growth and spread of the Christian influence in Europe. At that time, the church held nurses in high regard and made this known by bestowing sainthood on nursing leaders. Later, in the 16th century, secular trends in nursing began to evolve . . . [and] for more than three centuries after the Reformation, secular nursing carried with it no promise of a respectable career."[20]

Davis and Aroskar note that as late as the 1940s, nurses continued to be viewed in some ethics texts as servants of physicians and hospitals: "In 1943 . . . an author says that if the hospital hires the nurse, she is a servant of the hospital. . . . Any disobedience to the physician's orders is not only a matter of professional etiquette but a violation of the employee's contract."[21]

Nursing ethics can be characterized as a historical and continuing complexity of often competing allegiances, a struggle to reconcile Christian with secular values and to prioritize duties to patients, physicians, hospitals, nursing, self, society and to God. Today Leah Curtain speaks of nursing ethics in relation to the increasing institutionalization and bureaucratization of health care and the impact of moral pluralism.

"Nursing practice occurs within a context that involves a complex interaction of social and political values and certain relationships in society. Because of a particular mix of obligations impinging on nurses (as employees, employers, independent practitioners, patient advocates, physician extenders), nurses are frequently placed in paradoxical situations. . . . [Because of] the impact of moral pluralism . . . today there are debates about individual rights, societal rights and the responsibilities attached to these rights. . . . Society seems to be saying that freedom and self-determination are higher values than are health, and even life. . . . In today's health care system, individuals often cannot find a locus of authority."[22]

Many authors have cited reasons for the centrality and persistence of this dilemma within nursing. William Carpenter, for example, suggests that "nurses have been unable to exercise their competence in decision making and in patient care because they are locked into a role with extensive responsibility and limited authority."[23]

Dena Davis writes that nurses now argue for their status "as a profession distinct from but equal to medicine" and believes "it may be that nurses should also adopt different forms of ethical thinking." She highlights Carol Gilligan's work, expressing differences between male and female patterns of moral development.

"[Gilligan argues that] women tend to see human relationships from a different perspective than men; they emphasize relationality, caring and connectedness, while men emphasize rights, hierarchies and the boundaries between persons. Medicine [promotes] an ethic that focuses on individuation, respect for autonomy and rights in order to protect the weaker party in an unbalanced relationship. In contrast, the nursing profession, which . . . needs to . . . define itself as increasingly 'professional' without leaving behind the traditional values of care and comfort, may discover in contextual or narrative ethics the foundation for its identity."[24]

Curtain calls for nursing to redefine its ethics, based on a redefinition of itself. "The most pervasive ethical dilemma in nursing is that nurses are not free to practice nursing. . . . Nurses fill so many different roles and perform such radically different functions that a sociological definition of the profession is not possible. However, nursing can be, should be and is distinguished by its philosophy of care, its point of view and its particular approach to patients or clients. . . . The end or purpose of nursing is the well-being of other people. This end is not a scientific end; it is a moral end. That is, it involves the seeking of a good, and it involves relationships with other human beings. . . . *Nursing is a moral art.*"[25]

The values of caring, compassion and comfort seem to remain central to nursing within whatever context they may be expressed, but definitions shift; key values are exported from a biblical worldview and imposed in contexts where they remain ambiguous at best.

The dilemma of defining a locus of moral authority amid a prevailing moral pluralism is hardly unique to nursing; it is endemic within secular health care and society. And nursing, in seeking the type or essence of its ethics, consents to remain at the mercy of the ever-changing hit parade of fad values;

presently self-determination, empowerment and advocacy merit good press while servanthood, loyalty and vocation don't pull high ratings.

Journal of Christian Nursing editor Judy Shelly challenges Christian nurses to a biblical watchfulness and witness."The Christian mission of the Kaiserswerth deaconess community that nurtured and inspired Nightingale became lost in her desire for a 'secular order' of professional nurses. Is God restoring nursing to its Christian roots?. . . Let's keep our eyes on what God is doing [and] . . . as we perceive what God is doing, we must be willing to take risks, do new things and move into unknown territory, trusting God to lead the way. What would it mean to reclaim nursing for Jesus Christ?"[26]

Originally published in JCN, Spring, 1997

NOTES

1 Helen James, "Working for a Living: Judging the Border Collie, the Quintessential Blue-collar Dog," *AKC Gazette* (October 1995): 40.

2 M. Patricia Donahue, *Nursing, The Finest Art: An Illustrated History* (St. Louis: C. V. Mosby, 1985), p. 2.

3 Ibid., pp. 4-5.

4 Ibid., p. 11.

5 Ibid., p. 93.

6 Gerald Winslow, "From Loyalty to Advocacy: a New Metaphor for Nursing," *The Hastings Center Report* (June 1984): 32-33.

7 Isabel Robb, *Nursing Ethics for Hospital and Private Use* (Cleveland: E. C. Koeckert Pub., 1900), pp. 57, 60, 65.

8 Ibid., pp. 13-15.

9 Ibid., p. 65.

10 Ibid., p. 86.

11 Ibid., p. 33.

[12] Ibid., pp. 216-17.

[13] Ibid., pp. 252-58.

[14] M. Josephine Flaherty, "Nursing's Contract with Society," *Nursing Ethics: Theories and Pragmatics*, L. Curtin and M. J. Flaherty, eds. (Baltimore: Prentice-Hall Pub., 1982), p. 67.

[15] Ibid., p. 68.

[16] William Kilpatrick, "The Basis of Professional Ethics for Nurses," *American Journal of Nursing* 22, no. 10 (July 1922): 791.

[17] Diane Viens, "A History of the Code of Ethics for Nurses 1900-1985," *The Kansas Nurse* 64, no. 6: 5.

[18] Ibid.

[19] Ibid.

[20] Anne Davis and Mila Aroskar, *Ethical Dilemmas and Nursing Practice* (East Norwalk, Conn.: Appleton and Lange, 1991), pp. 53-54.

[21] Ibid., p. 55.

[22] Leah Curtain, "The Nurse-Patient Relationship: Foundation, Purposes, Responsibilities and Rights," *Nursing Ethics: Theories and Pragmatics*, L. Curtain and M. J. Flaherty, eds. (Baltimore: Prentice-Hall Pub., 1982), pp. 81-83.

[23] William Carpenter, "Nursing," *Encyclopedia of Bioethics* 3, Warren Reich, ed. (New York: The Free Press, 1978), p. 1140.

[24] Dena Davis, "Nursing: An Ethic of Caring," *Humane Medicine* 2, no. 1 (1983): 21, 25.

[25] Curtain, "Nurse-Patient Relationship," pp. 85-86.

[26] Judith Shelly, "Living with Change," *Journal of Christian Nursing* 13, no. 1 (Winter 1996): 36.

29

Disability in the Body of Christ

Linda L. Treloar

Why do some significantly disabled people respond bitterly, while others seem resilient despite continuing adversity? As a nurse and the mother of a severely disabled adult child, I began to wonder why some people with disabilities seem to have a bitter root (see Hebrews 12:15) that permeates their spirits, coloring their response to life, its meaning and their relationships. However, I saw others with serious limitations whose lives are filled with joy.

My question and experiences led me to explore the relationships between spiritual beliefs, response to disability and the evangelical Christian church's influence on people affected by disability. In 1998 I interviewed thirty people, including nine adults with physical disabilities and thirteen parents of disabled children, living in a Southwestern metropolitan area.[1] The participants, nearly all Caucasians with a variety of denominational and nondenominational religious backgrounds, ascribe to evangelical Christian beliefs.

My faith grew as I listened to the participants tell stories involving trial and hardship, while expressing thankfulness to God and choosing to live with joy. Each expressed a belief in God's greater purpose and plan for his or her life. Both parents and adults with disabilities experienced God in ordinary and extraordinary events of life. Trials or difficulty contributed to spiritual challenge, the breaking of self-centeredness, reliance on God and strengthened faith. The participants' spiritual beliefs stabilized their lives, providing meaning for the experience of disability, assistance with coping and many other benefits.

The study contributes to the growing body of knowledge that establishes a positive role for religious faith in experiences that affect well-being. While solid support by the church promoted positive adaptation to disability, it was not as important as the participants' personal relationship with Jesus Christ. The study produced rich findings for people concerned about the church and families affected by disability. Likewise, the participants have much to teach health professionals about spiritual health and well-being.

Applications for Health Professionals

We all seek answers for difference (disability), suffering and illness. Christian health professionals can provide support to people affected by disabilities and guidance to church leaders and congregations. Two biblical imperatives underlie our actions: love for God and love for one another (see Matthew 22:37-40). We must ask, "What does it mean to live as the body of Christ today? How does this influence our personal and professional practice as disabled and non-disabled persons in Christian community?"

Health professionals *who accompany people on their journey* with disability are sorely needed. Deeply listening to people's stories can promote spiritual well-being for them and you. I heard accounts of difficulty and relief, frustration and satisfaction, sorrow and joy.

At the end of his family's interview, Ted, a minister, said, "I think there's healing just in talking about this today." A few weeks later, he chose not to review the family's *portrait*, a summary of their conversation and its main themes. His wife, Marg, explained that in day-to-day life, "Denial is used as a coping mechanism, but when our story is written in front of us, reality can't be avoided." Though a degree of healing was achieved for Ted, it was still in process.

Spiritual challenge appears understandable: why would a good God give these parents a child with disabilities since they sought his direction and had made a commitment for pastoral ministry? Their life circumstances were incongruent with their spiritual beliefs about God's will for their lives. Nearly eighteen years later, Ted continues to struggle with spiritual challenge and guilt, as his ability to discern God's will for his life and that of others has been shaken. Adaptation to disability exists alongside chronic sorrow.

Disability poses the general problem of natural evil: could—and, if so, should—God not have created the world in a way that such accidents did not occur?[2] Lacking theological explanations, the public may view God as not good, as a "meanie in the sky."

Bill, a parent who attended mainline Protestant churches or a non-denominational Bible church on a regular basis for more than forty years, expresses his frustration: "What does the Bible say about the disabled? I assume nothing because I've never heard anything. I'm certain I'm wrong. What did Jesus say about the disabled? Are there any references? I don't know. I would assume no. That makes it difficult even for Christians to rectify that and to justify disability in their minds. If the pastor never preaches anything about the disabled, then my thought is that Jesus never addressed the issue. I know he healed the disabled—don't get me wrong. But how does Jesus hear them? Are they special? Are they different? I would guess that, but I have no biblical background to back that up."

Lack of a biblical foundation for finding meaning in disability promoted spiritual distress and movement away from God and the church for a few participants. Bill believes that his lack of a biblical foundation for understanding disability allowed Satan to tempt him years earlier with thoughts that God was punishing him by withholding miraculous healing for his daughter, Cathy. Bill, like others, did not understand why God does not always heal.

The public, in general, and people affected by disability need clearly articulated information to help them establish a theological basis for meaning surrounding these issues.

Barry speaks from personal experience with physical disabilities and from his perspective as a counselor of people with disabilities and of their families. He observes patterns of blame in others—toward self, spouse or God. Barry explains, "I see a lot of families breakup because a child is disabled. The mother will blame the father, too, sometimes. The blame has to be put somewhere. They either put it on each other, or they put it on God: 'God did this to us; why did he?' Men do not like to accept failure. Basically, if they fail in the seed they plant, and the child is not the perfect child, they feel they've failed. It's hard for a man to say, 'I did that. It's because of me.' Most are in denial. Men do not open up; they do not talk about things. The first thing they're *not* going to say is, 'My son's crippled or disabled.'"

In the same vein, when Theresa's multiply-disabled son was born, she said, "I thought God was punishing me. I couldn't believe it! I really had a rough time. I didn't understand how God could give me a problem like this, when I had so many problems already."

Why do *bad* or inconvenient things like disability happen to *good* people? Does God create disabilities? What did I do to deserve this? Why doesn't God heal me (or my loved one)? Do I lack faith? Many participants questioned why God allowed difficulty in their lives. This reflects spiritual challenge and the need to establish meaning for disability. However, blaming and questioning God appeared to be separate, but overlapping, issues.

Unfortunately, no single answers exist for these questions, even within the same religious tradition.[3] The problem is magnified with lack of clear or adequate biblical teaching.[4] In the midst of theological confusion and public attitudes surrounding the meaning of disability, people with disabilities may internalize negative messages. The outcome may be rejection of God and spiritual beliefs that could be helpful.[5] I strongly recommend that churches openly address these issues from a scriptural perspective so that church leaders and the congregation alike have a theological basis for establishing meaning related to disability.

Health professionals need to become familiar with theological explanations for questions surrounding disability, suffering, sin, healing and adequacy of faith.

Jim, traumatically injured as a young adult, remarked that well-meaning Christians failed to provide helpful, biblically-based counsel. He commented, "Christians would come to visit me in the hospital, and most would have some answer. They'd say, 'I feel this or that about your accident. This is why it happened. God has a reason for these things.' It was not comforting to have somebody say that God has a reason for this, when you're in the middle of it. One pastor said, 'For every non-Christian who has an injury or an accident, God puts a Christian through the same sort of ordeal to show the world the difference.'

"I said, 'No! Just stop! I know you're trying to help, but that isn't any help at all. Let's not waste time on things that might be true, but you don't know are true—because you don't know.' The things that God said to us in the Bible were the only things that were true, helpful and nurturing to me."

The participants' experiences with disability influenced their relationship with God: they desired a closer, personal relationship with Jesus and biblically-based support and counsel by Christians. Health professionals who effectively minister to people affected by disability and their families provide a spiritually sensitive presence that doesn't need to offer answers to disability. However, when counsel is given in response to the client's or family's request for direction, it should be based on scriptural truth. Professionals who offer such spiritual support can be effective role models for family and church leaders.

Since becoming the parent of a daughter with disabilities, Ted said, "What has grown for me is compassion—being more sensitive to people who are disabled or not as attractive in mind or body. . . When I was in grade school, I was one of those jerks who was mean to kids that couldn't keep up. I've had to do some major rethinking about that. God is a God of concern for everybody, not just people who are 100 percent physical, 100 percent mental, 100 percent anything."

Wanted: Compassion, Not Pity

A recurring theme involves the participants' desire to be treated with compassion rather than with pity. Both adults with disabilities and family members described a deep pain associated with the experience of disability that others cannot or do not choose to share.

Mary commented that she feels lonely when her son, Paul, is hospitalized, despite the presence of visitors. She remains isolated; people hold themselves back from participating in her pain. Mary says, "Every time Paul's been in the hospital, that's the most lonesome time with everybody around me. I feel like saying, 'What are you all doing? Where is your concern?' It's like they're putting on a facade: 'We did our thing. We came and visited and said our prayers. But, I could feel them saying, 'Don't let me get too close for fear I'll hurt.'"

Both Jim and his wife, Angela, complained about others' lack of understanding of their suffering following his spinal cord injury. Yet Angela found that she, similar to others, was unexplainably blocked from showing compassion to Jim. One day in the hospital, his body lay at an angle that resembled the bodies of geriatric patients she had cared for in the past. This revolted her. Angela's personal response to the physical changes in Jim still trouble her, eighteen months after his accident. She says, "I was totally revolted by the whole thing. I felt so guilty. Talk about having no compassion! We talk about all those people who had no compassion for us. I didn't have compassion for Jim. And I still don't, to a certain degree. It's like there's a part of my heart that can't come to grips. Something inhibits me from showing compassion to Jim. He wants me to rub his legs. I don't have the compassion to do it. That's terrible. It bothers me greatly. Of course, he can't understand why. Really, I don't either."

Too often, others respond not out of compassion but out of pity. Yet Angela, strangely enough, experienced the same reservations in serving Jim that the participants complained about.

Robert F. Murphy in *The Body Silent* notes, "The disabled person's radical bodily difference, his departure from the human standard, dominates the thoughts of the other and may even repel him. But these are thoughts that can barely be articulated, let alone voiced."[6] What is it about disability that affronts our psyche and our spirit, that stops us from serving one another and changes our relationships? What is it that prohibits us from seeing disability as difference, rather than as something abnormal?

Cathy, a young adult with disabilities, suggests that the core issue is whether or not meaning for disability has been established, regardless of spiritual or religious beliefs. She observes that more Christians than non-Christians have failed to reach some level of meaning about disability, but she cannot explain why this is the case. Based on the data, I suggest that theological confusion over sin, disability and related issues must be considered.

When Jim was hospitalized after his accident, the most helpful health care professionals were those who asked his opinion; they invited his participation in his care. He contrasted the actions and attitude of a nurse who demonstrated compassion toward him with those whom he perceived as patronizing. He says, "When she came into the room, she treated me as a person, as an adult, as a twenty-nine-year-old male, as a peer. She had to do everything for me: clean me up, brush my teeth—whatever. But that's how she treated me.

"At the other extreme are the people who patronized me, who would just as soon give me a pill and put me out as they would extend themselves to help me. Nights and weekends were the worst. There were two nurses whom I dreaded. It was a nightmare to have them come in. Then there are the people who would never leave me alone, who mothered me to death."

The first nurse maintained Jim's worth and value as a peer and saw his physical limitations as incidental, not primary. The others belittled him: he took on the role of a child, while they acted as parents. These nurses exemplify the difference between compassion and pity toward Jim. *Compassion maintains the person's worth; pity offers help while it squashes the recipient's self.*

Caregivers Need A Break

Participants repeatedly recommended that churches designate people to gather information on specific needs of this population. Parents would like for churches to ask directly, "What do you need?" and offer periods of caregiving. Parents commonly complained about *fighting* to meet their children's needs during the week. They are unlikely to attend church if this pattern continues on the seventh day. The data support the idea that people with disabilities have needs that are common to others, yet unique (the same, but different).

Marg explains, "If I could make a suggestion to churches, I think the greatest need would have been for them to come to me and ask, 'What can I do to help you?' And second, to offer to take Beth, sometimes, so that the rest of our family could do something together that we were hindered from doing with her, like playing games, just normal games, for instance, that we had to lay down (becoming tearful), or time for Ted and me. It made us work to ask for help with Beth.

"It's hard to ask. The first and second time you feel like maybe people won't mind. But the fifth year and the twelfth year and the fourteenth year, I hesitated and felt like people started avoiding me for fear they'd have to help. I felt like my presence made people feel guilty. I sensed people backing away from me. A child grows up. You get babysitters for a short while. But with a child with disabilities, you still need the relief. You still need the help."

Marg's pain was obvious as she described the difficulty of asking for help from others. She raises the need for respite care and the importance of addressing the population with an extended rather than a limited perspective. As the years passed, she observed others backing away from her, avoiding her.

Health professionals can serve the body of Christ by assessing for needs and advocating for people affected by disability. Parish nurses are ideally positioned to assist others in ministry to and with this population. Serving people with disabilities includes an ability to know what to do, along with action that conveys sensitivity, awareness and acceptance of these families.

A few participants noted the common perception that people with ordinary skills cannot meet the needs of this population. Monica takes Jenny, who uses a power wheelchair, to church. She refutes this notion and says, "It's a compassion thing. It's an action, not just talking or feeling sorry. It is hard! It is a sacrifice! God's touching people to do this. Very few people are willing. People are so wound up in their own problems, but their problems would probably diminish if they would step out and help somebody else."

Jeff complained that it's difficult to educate churches, like health professionals, about the needs of people with disabilities. While professionals "don't listen," he felt that churches "don't care." Churches verbalize a concern and interest but fail to provide effective help and lack understanding of the population's needs. This conveys a problem with attitudinal accessibility. Jeff says, "I think what Connie and I both found is that the churches are the hardest group to educate. You could go to the doctors and say, 'This is what is going on with Aaron and his needs.' They won't listen. The churches say, 'Okay, okay, okay.' They don't care. They try to. They talk a good talk. But when it comes down to it, they say, 'We can't do that.' Why? That's what you're here for. Most people are not exposed to disabilities, either physical or mental. They don't know what to do, how to act. They don't know what to do because they don't understand what the family's needs are."

Jeff's comment that churches don't understand the needs of families with disabilities was echoed by nearly all of the participants. Both parents and adults with disabilities frequently acknowledged the Christian community's lack of service to one another, even apart from that to the disabled community. I suggest that health professionals with varied backgrounds should join disabled persons and their families in educating churches and others on the needs and resources available to people affected by disability.

Angela said that churches should relate to people with disabilities as whole persons, recognizing that physical needs may dominate this population's view and focus. She says, "People with disabilities appear different than we (non-disabled) are. But they're just like us. The only thing that separates us from them is physical needs that can come and press in on a person so strongly that it can almost be the only world they know. That need can crush them. That need dominates their total existence. That need is ever-present, without relief. You need to find a way as ministers through the church to be with them as people, just like we are; but, at the same time, you need to recognize the intensity and all-consuming nature of their physical spirit being. You have to minister to the whole person."

Angela accurately describes the domination of physical needs on one's being, creating an "ever-present need, without relief." Acknowledging a whole being, consisting of mind, body and spirit, influences one's relationships with the population. Health professionals who fail to integrate spiritual care considerations into health care practice miss their greatest opportunity for service to others.

Several participants agreed that one of the best ways to help meet people's needs is for churches to provide a mechanism for the networking of families and resources in the community, such as through a small group. Karen says, "Families drop out of churches due to lack of support and lack of hearing about other similar families in their church. In other words, the Johnson family has a disabled child, and the Smith family has one, as well. Those two families can link up. There's not enough of that."

Health professionals could readily lead networking efforts and provide effective referral guidance to the population. Most participants agreed, however, that it is unlikely that families will ask for such assistance. It has typically not been available, and a majority of the participants don't expect the church to minister to them in this way.

A few participants reported that pastors, similar to their parishioners, don't know how to relate to people with disabilities: they don't understand the disability experience. Kevin, a former Catholic priest and a mental health counselor, says, "Most pastors can go in and talk to families about dying, but they can't talk about living with disability." He believes that churches should join together to provide qualified counselors, who are sensitive to and specifically trained in disability issues. Cathy believes that counsel should be provided to children apart from their parents, so parents' needs and beliefs don't interfere with those of their children. Further, church staff should *initiate* this kind of ministry contact.

Several participants verbalized awareness that people with disabilities are greatly underrepresented in churches. They suggest that reasons for this include faulty assumptions about the needs of the participants, lack of knowledge of disability by others, discomfort with disabilities and avoidance by church staff. Other reasons stated include excessive caregiving stresses by families and churches unprepared to integrate the population into the congregation. Although they admit that disability may contribute to fear and avoidance by those who do not share the experience, they believe the solution begins with serving one another. Although the population has gifts to share with others, they may be viewed as a burden or a drain on limited personnel and resources.

In a Nutshell

The participants are social beings, deeply affected by the experience of living with disability. Adaptation occurred within the context of relationships with God and others. What the participants believe influenced how they live: spiritual beliefs stabilized their lives. They chose to live in joy with thankfulness, despite ongoing difficulty, and to be used by God to help others.

John says, "My faith has to do with filling me with joy. If I'm filled with joy, and I think of joyous things, I don't think about what would embitter me, regardless of my physical limitations —and they are many. My faith, quite literally, has kept me alive. Without something stable to hold onto, I don't think I would have made it. Without faith, I probably would have committed suicide."

The challenge is ours: what does it mean to live as the body of Christ? People with disabilities can achieve spiritual balance and strength with the help of caring health professionals who assist families to grapple with spiritual issues related to disability and move toward positive theological understanding of the meaning of the experience.

Originally published in JCN, Summer, 2000

NOTES

[1] Linda L. Treloar, "Perceptions of Spiritual Beliefs, Responses to Disability and the Church," (PhD Diss., The Union Institute, 1999).

[2] David A. Pailin, *A Gentle Touch: From a Theology of Handicap to a Theology of Human Being* (London: SPCK, 1992), p. 42.

[3] George W. Paterson, *Helping Your Handicapped Child* (Minneapolis: Augsburg Publishing House, 1975).

[4] William Blair and Dana Davidson, "To the Glory of God: *Hesed,* Hospitality and Disabilities," in *And Show Steadfast Love,* Lewis H. Merrick, ed. (Louisville, Ky.: Presbyterian Church, 1993), pp. 7-28; William A. Blair, "Ministry to Persons with Disabilities: Can We Do Better?" *Journal of Religion in Disability and Rehabilitation* 1, no. 1 (1994): 1-9.

[5] Nancy L. Eiesland, *The Disabled God: Toward a Liberatory Theology of Disability* (Nashville, Tenn.: Abingdon Press, 1994).

[6] Charles Gourgey, "Enlarge the Site of Your Tent: Making a Place in the Church for People with Disabilities," in *And Show Steadfast Love,* Lewis H. Merrick, ed. (Louisville, Ky.: Presbyterian Church, 1993), pp. 29-45.

30

Breaking the Cycle of School Violence

Joyce E. Peterson

Violence is *the* issue in schools today because of the increasing number of shooting incidents. Since the shootings at Columbine High School, school officials, staff, parents and students live in fear of what might happen in their own school. They are rightly concerned with safety and the prevention of violence, for violence continues to threaten our schools. I began to think about the reasons our youth exhibited so much violence and wondered if parish nurses could make a difference. Could parish nurses help reduce the violence? I believe that we can do that, not only in schools but in the community in general.

First, parish nurses are concerned with and promote the health of the whole person: physical, mental, emotional and spiritual. In addition, they are committed to the prevention and early identification of illness. Violence is an illness, reaching epidemic proportions in our society. It is an illness that keeps us asking why it is happening and what we can do about it. It is an illness that screams loudly for treatment.

It would be wise to ask if violence is really on the rise or if it is simply getting more press now, since there are those who insist this is the case. *Preventing Youth Handgun Violence: A National Study with Trends and Patterns for the State of Colorado* reports that "Handgun homicides committed by young males (age 15-18) between 1980 and 1995 increased by more than 150 percent."[1]

The website "School Violence—Let's Get It Out of Our System" reports several research and survey findings. Among these findings is the fact that the percent of students reporting street gang presence at school nearly doubled between 1989 and 1995. In addition, the percentage of elementary teachers who say students disrupt the classroom most of the time or fairly often has increased from 48 percent in 1984 to 65 percent in 1997.[2] Numerous other findings are reported, giving evidence to much threatening and violent behavior in our schools. Although the latter findings are not compared with earlier findings and cannot prove that violence is on the increase, they do indicate that violence exists in alarming proportions.

My personal observations as a school nurse have convinced me that violence is increasing and that more and more children are able to cope with unpleasant events in their lives only in a violent manner. The number of playground fights, threats toward other students or teachers, incidents of verbal abuse and weapons brought to school is definitely on the increase and is alarming to both students and staff. We live in a rural area where discipline, respect and parental cooperation are the norm, but we see less and less of these positive behaviors and more and more negative behaviors, including violence, as each year passes.

Violence, whether on the increase or not, is an illness in our society. It is an illness that most people want to eradicate and one that has received much attention lately with a variety of theories about what to do about it. With so many people already working on the problem, is there a need for parish nurses to get involved? My answer is a resounding *yes*.

What Causes Violence?

There is no one easy answer, but several components have been identified as contributing to a violent attitude and violent behavior. Lorel Fox cites a Gallup poll that lists factors young people believe contribute to a climate of violence, including peer pressure, a lack of adult respect for teens, physical abuse, too much television, feelings of alienation, missing parents (through divorce or death), dangerous music and risky behavior.[3]

J. H. Laub and J. L. Lauritsen connect violence with certain social conditions, stating, "Violent behavior is the product of the interaction between individual development and social contexts (e.g., the family, school and neighborhood)."[4] They cite several factors contributing to violence including low socioeconomic status, high population turnover, race and ethnicity, single-parent households and high housing density. They also state, "These conditions lower a neighborhood's capacity for social organization and its ability to exert informal social control."[5]

When I was a child, my parents knew all our neighbors and the parents of all my friends. No matter where I was, someone who knew my parents was watching out for me and willing to report my behavior. These informal social controls helped keep my friends and me on the straight and narrow path, not only because someone was watching but also because someone cared. This, to me, is what is meant by the often-quoted statement, "It takes a village to raise a child."

Today we don't know our neighbors. We are so busy with work that we often don't belong to many social groups and consequently don't get acquainted with people who could be our neighbors. People often feel isolated, alone and convinced that because no one cares how they behave, it really doesn't matter. The lack of both formal and informal social organization is a contributing factor to violence.

These factors often lead children to form their own social organizations known as gangs, which usually react violently to nearly any provocation. Many of the factors that the young people say contribute to violence are likely to be a direct result of the social disorganization. Lack of respect often stems from not knowing the people who live nearby. Peer pressure and feelings of alienation are often reduced when adults in addition to parents are present and caring.

Breaking the Cycle

To break the cycle of violence, we need to concentrate on reaching the children. If young men have not committed a violent act by the time they reach eighteen or twenty-one, it is highly unlikely that they ever will. Dr. Delbert Elliott, of the Task Force for the Study and Prevention of Violence at the University of Colorado at Boulder, states that those who are out of control or exhibit violent tendencies in early childhood are likely to have serious problems later.[6] Therefore, it seems, we must reach the children.

On the other hand, in the case of behavior, we must reach and help the parents as well. Children tend to imitate their parents' values, whether they admit it or not. Parents are a strong influence on their children, and children want their parents to teach them, to share their ideas, their thoughts and their feelings. Therefore, it is important to help parents.

The most difficult period for children is between the ages of eleven and seventeen. As children get older, they must function not only in the family but in social situations with their peers. A strong, stable and loving family life will help children face such situations with confidence. A lack of such family influence will contribute to behavioral problems and violence. Helping families know how to become a part of an organized social situation will go a long way toward stopping the violence we are experiencing today.

Many ideas have surfaced about how to stem violence. I think some well-meaning people are on the wrong track. Some groups are mounting a major effort to ban guns in one way or another. Many people believe that getting rid of guns will decrease violence, since guns have been used in much of the violence that has occurred. On June 16, 1997, Vice President Gore announced that 6,276 students had been expelled for bringing weapons to school during the 1995-96 school year and declared that this showed that President Clinton's efforts to make schools safer were working. The Gun-Free Schools Act made a zero-tolerance policy against guns in schools mandatory. "Today, the numbers are in, and [the] message is clear: there's no place for guns or violence in America's schools," the former vice president said.[7] The shootings at Columbine High occurred in 1998.

I don't believe in allowing guns at school, but I don't think the zero-tolerance policy will stop violence. It may go some distance to stop shootings, but it won't stop the anger, the lack of connection or the feelings of isolation that contribute to violence. It will simply allow those feelings to be shown in some other violent way. Why did the students who were expelled bring guns in the first place? Did they intend violence, or were they trying to protect themselves from violence someone might commit against them? It might not be clear thinking, but immature thinkers may not make wise decisions. It is important to prevent the situations that bring about such decisions by students.

Other suggestions to prevent violence include a variety of ways to increase security at schools. Nearly every school district has developed a plan to follow in the event of a bomb threat, a shooter or the threat of any other violent act. The plans include tip boxes; identification cards for students and staff, with sign-in and passes for visitors; frequent rounds by law enforcement officers and locked doors. Some schools have installed fences and metal detectors.[8]

Most of these solutions are like waiting until a disease hits and then giving gamma globulin and hoping it works, instead of getting immunized before being exposed. These things don't cure the underlying cause of the violence; rather, they just try to stop it from happening, probably only postponing it, or they punish it more severely. While I certainly believe in punishing those who do violence, I believe strongly in trying to prevent it in the first place.

Another solution frequently mentioned is getting students involved in the prevention of violence with things like tip boxes, dress codes, stopping or reporting harassment and treating one another with respect. One group is advocating the use of athletes as models in this new behavior. Some experts proposed talking to football coaches throughout Colorado since the Columbine shooting, encouraging them to enlist the help of athletes in stopping the harassment of other students and modeling tolerance toward all. Jackson Katz says that athletes enjoy status as leaders in schools and should be encouraged to help.[9] Unfortunately, after the Columbine shootings, some students complained that athletes formed a powerful clique and often harassed other students.

One day I walked into the second-grade room to talk to a student just as the teacher was conducting the character education lesson for the day. She was talking to the class and using role playing to help students learn how to deal with others who are bullying or threatening them. "Kids who are threatening, pressuring and intimidating you don't have a good self-image," she said. "They are trying to make themselves feel better by putting themselves in a position of power."

If she is correct, and I believe she is, then why are athletes, who enjoy status and should be feeling powerful already, harassing and intimidating other students? Apparently, many students have low self-esteem, and being powerful isn't necessarily solving their problem. Obviously, other underlying needs must also be met for them to feel good about themselves. I believe it is important to help students learn how to treat one another, but I have two concerns about a project like this. First, power can be dangerous in the hands of students with low self-esteem. We could be unleashing monsters, if we keep emphasizing the power these athletes have over others. They may hear only the part about power and fail to listen to the part about responsibility. These are, after all, immature youth. Second, the responsibility may be too much. Giving students responsibility for helping prevent violence must be carefully handled, or the guilt could be overwhelming if serious violence occurs, especially the loss of life.

Dr. Elliott reports that programs that target the individual such as tip lines, identification cards, gun buybacks, and even the DARE programs, don't succeed.[10] So, what works? According to Elliott, prenatal home visits to young, low-income women expecting their first child have been effective. These visits reduced abuse, drug use rates and delinquency. What an opportunity for parish nurses to impact the future behavior of our youth! We can do that.

Shay Bilchik, a Justice Department official, stated, "Pulling our community together . . . is the fundamental basis of a violence-reduction program."[11] He went on to say that reducing violence isn't complicated, but it does require involvement of everyone in the community. I felt that he was also saying that it takes a village to raise a child. He is not saying that the parents don't have primary responsibility, but he is saying that the community needs to work together to set expectations and to give support when and where it is needed. This is another way that parish nurses can help promote the conditions that lead to the reduction of violence.

M. A. Hamburg says that although violence has been seen as a problem of the judicial and social fields, a public health approach has become an increasingly important resource, since it emphasizes prevention by identifying risk factors and taking steps to educate about and protect against them. "The public health approach allows one to think about violence not as an inevitable fact of life but as a problem that can be prevented. It empowers individuals and communities to reduce the risk factors leading to violent behavior," according to Hamburg.[12] Education and prevention are two major aspects of the parish nurse's job. Certainly we can have an impact here.

What Can You Do?

What practical steps can the parish nurse take to help reduce violence among school-age children? Certainly the prenatal visits to any mother expecting her first child can be of great benefit, with an emphasis on low-income families, especially single women. However, a spiritual assessment of every expectant mother and efforts to meet those needs, as well as the physical needs, will certainly improve the results. Referrals to agencies that can help the mother meet her needs has been shown to be effective and is part of the parish nurse's realm of authority.

The parish nurse can match families in need with helpers. Finding a surrogate grandparent for a young family can go a long way toward avoiding feelings of alienation, isolation or that no one is paying attention. Facilitating a mentoring program can do the same thing for individual children in need of a caring adult role model. A Parents Teaching Parents program would be another way to match people in need with those who have skills to share.

Through these programs, the parish nurse can also help the congregation see that in areas of high housing-density, the church can be the social organization small enough to watch out for the individual or family. Starting early in a child's life to provide a strong social support system is important. If a child reaches eleven feeling that he needs a social group to take the place of his family, he is more likely to join a gang.

Parish nurses can organize educational programs that would be extremely helpful in reducing violence, such as programs that teach children how to deal with bullies or those who taunt or exhibit threatening behavior. Adult educational programs could focus on parenting skills that increase a child's self-esteem.

Organizing a volunteer program for youth in the church would go a long way toward reducing violence. Volunteerism helps youth gain respect from adults and reduces feelings of alienation. It also gets them away from the TV and builds self-esteem by giving youth an opportunity to serve others.

At the same time, youth get acquainted with more people in the community, increasing the opportunity for networking and social organization. People who work in the community usually take pride in it and are less likely to commit violence against it. Knowing that others in the community are watching and caring also reduces risky behavior.

The parish nurse cannot and should not do it all. However, we can and should have a major impact on reducing violence among our children through the programs we implement and oversee, especially if we are centered in Christ and dedicated to doing his will. Proverbs 4:13 reminds us, "Keep hold of instruction; do not let go; guard her, for she is your life." Verse 18 goes on to say, "But the path of the righteous is like the light of dawn, which shines brighter and brighter until full day."

Sunlight usually makes people feel better, more positive, more alive and better able to face the day. The sunlight of the parish nurse can bring an attitude of confidence and hope to the lives we touch and to those for whom we provide knowledge and care.

Originally published in JCN, Summer, 2000

NOTES

1 Center for the Study and Prevention of Violence (1999). *CSPV Fact Sheet.* On-line. Available http://www.colorado.edu/cspv/fact sheets/factsheet16.html.

[2] *School Violence: Let's Get It Out of Our System* (1998). On-line. Available http://www2.cnsu.edu/ncsu/cep/PreViolence/eoto98.htm.

[3] Gallup poll, cited in Lorel K. Fox, "Contributing to Violence," *The Lutheran* (November 1999): 58.

[4] Center for the Study and Prevention of Violence (1999). *CSPV Fact Sheet*. On-line. Available http://www.colorado.edu/cspv/fact sheets/factsheet6.html.

[5] Ibid.

[6] Peter G. Chronis, "Patterns of Violent Behavior Cited," *The Denver Post* (August 28, 1999). On-line. Available http://www.denver-post.com/news/shot0828.htm.

[7] Albert Gore, *White House Release* (June 16, 1997). On-line. Available http://www.cyfc.umn.edu/Learn/press/061697.html.

[8] Chronis.

[9] Neil H. Devlin, "Recruit Athletes to Foil Violence, Coaches Are Told," *The Denver Post* (August 11, 1999). Available http://www.den verpost.com/news/shot0811.htm.

[10] Chronis.

[11] Students' Reports on School Crime, 1989 and 1995, *National Center for Education Statistics Bureau of Justice Statistics* (1998). On-line. Available http://www2.ncsu.edu/ncsu/cep/PreViolence/eoto98.htm.

[12] Center for the Study and Prevention of Violence, 1999. *CSPV Fact Sheet*. On-line. Available http://www.colorado.edu/cspv/factsheets /factsheet9.html.

31

Adolescent Sexual Crises

Jeffery J. McNeil

Fifteen-year-old Sara and her mother came to the ambulatory care clinic for a problem defined only as personal. During the initial interview, Sara expressed interest in birth control. Her mother interrupted, "I caught her having sex. I want her put on the pill. The last thing she needs is a baby."

Various concerns flooded my mind as I listened to their story. Current nursing literature confirms what most would suspect: sexually transmitted diseases and unwanted pregnancy are prevalent among Sara's age group. Her mother probably felt somewhat isolated in her attempt to help Sara and desperate to prevent long-term problems. Sara's spiritual well-being was not mentioned, so I knew nothing about the family's religious faith. Nevertheless, I was committed to meeting the needs of Sara and her mother on a physical, social and spiritual level, and planned to discuss each one.

Sara's mother had reason for concern. Current statistical information shows Sara is not alone. Sexual activity among high-school youth has practically doubled in the past twenty years. A recent survey indicates that 66 percent of females and 67.1 percent of males are sexually active by their senior year in high school. Twenty-five percent of high-school males and 21 percent of the females have experienced four or more sexual partners.[1] With this increasing sexual activity, over the last decade the U.S. has witnessed an epidemic of sexually transmitted diseases (STDs) and one of the highest teen pregnancy rates in the Western world. American youth are in trouble. Sara's mother was surprised to learn this and responded, "Things were sure different in my day."

The 1970s brought a transformation in sexual thinking: the touting of *free love* and self-satisfaction, with little regard for consequences. It was a time of questioning authority, including the Bible as the absolute standard for behavior. The rejection of absolutes left individuals free to determine their own fluctuating value systems. Since the 1970s, we have witnessed family demise, as the divorce rate has quadrupled from 4.3 million in 1970 to 17.4 million in 1994.[2] Children are too often without their mother and father in the home, causing many youth to turn to friends for support and guidance in life issues, for which the peers are ill prepared.

Pregnancy and STDs

The only positive trend in our humanistic efforts to decrease teen pregnancy is the rate decline from 1990 to 1995.[3] Effective methods of contraception have been available in private practice and family planning clinics throughout the U.S. Unfortunately, this will not protect Sara from sexually transmitted diseases. Three million new cases of STDs occur each year in teens. Chlamydia is detected in 10 to 29 percent of sexually active female adolescents, while the human papilloma virus is detected in 15 percent of them. Gonorrhea is found in 1 to 5 percent of sexually active female adolescents and is higher among teens than any other age group.[4]

The human immunodeficiency virus (HIV) is also a problem in adolescents. Twenty percent of people diagnosed in their twenties were infected during adolescence. Adolescent AIDS cases increased 77 percent from 1990 to 1992.[5] HIV climbs as the seventh leading cause of death among females between fifteen and twenty-four, with heterosexual activity responsible for 50 percent of cases.[6]

In addition to STDs, adolescent pregnancy can lead to many other problems. Sixty-two percent of pregnant teens drop out of high school.[7] Teen mothers are less likely to get married and more likely to receive public assistance than those who do not get pregnant. Most teens' fetuses never make it to delivery; 43 percent are aborted. This statistic may increase to 92 percent among the more affluent.[8] The infants carried to term still face many disadvantages: they are more likely to drop out of school and end up on welfare, creating a cycle of poverty. They often become part of our criminal justice system. Who pays for these sins? The American public puts up approximately $29 billion a year in increased education, welfare and prison expense.[9] If Sara is fortunate enough to escape pregnancy, she still faces an enemy that can destroy her present and future.

Gonorrhea is the most frequently reported sexually transmitted disease in the U.S. Seventy-five percent of women who have it have no symptoms to indicate they are infected.[10] The absence of symptoms has also skyrocketed chlamydia, a virus-like bacteria, to America's most common STD. Many infected persons are unaware that they are passing along this disease during a sexual encounter. It can result in infection of the epididymis and prostate gland in men, and the uterus, fallopian tubes and ovaries in women, often leading to infertility in both sexes.

"If not adequately treated, 20 to 40 percent of women infected with chlamydia and 10 to 40 percent of women with gonorrhea develop upper genital tract infection, also called pelvic inflammatory disease (PID). Among women with PID, scarring will result in infertility in 20 percent, potentially fatal ectopic pregnancy in 9 percent and chronic pelvic pain in 18 percent."[11] Other sequelae may include rectal abscesses, heart disease and meningitis.

The herpes simplex virus and human papilloma virus (HPV) can also have a significant impact on teens. Herpes simplex can lead to central nervous system problems ranging from pain to meningitis, or cause chronic cervicitis. Currently, there is no cure, which explains why one of every five adults over twenty-five is infected.[12] The human papilloma virus has 120 types, many of which cause genital warts. Approximately two-thirds of exposed partners will become infected.[13] HPV is now believed to be a leading cause of abnormal pap smears and cervical cancer.

These are only four of the many sexual diseases that threaten youth like Sara. With so much information available, Sara's mother asked why young people continue on such destructive paths.

Developmental Problems

Adolescents begin sexual maturation as early as twelve, while cognitive abilities lag behind. In their struggle to discover who they are as individuals, teens are strongly influenced by external forces. Peer and family relationships may either build or threaten self-esteem. Menarche occurs earlier today than a hundred years ago, the average age dropping two years to an all-time low of 12.5 years. The hormonal influence brings a sexual awakening that a child is not emotionally prepared to handle. Sexually explicit TV programs bombard the consciousness, which can lead to the belief that *everybody is doing it.* Teens use alcohol and drugs as stress outlets, decreasing their ability to make rational decisions. Morality and values are seldom discussed by health care professionals. After all, who has the right to tell someone else what is right and wrong? The decision is left to the individual—a tall order for a fifteen-year-old.

According to Swiss psychologist Jean Piaget's theory of cognitive development, teens are not fully developed in operational thinking, which is essential for planning for the future. Since they do not connect present actions with future results, practicing preventive behavior is difficult for them. Another cognitive characteristic of adolescence is *magical thinking*,[14] the belief that the individual is protected from danger that comes to others. Most people can recall activities they participated in as teens but would never consider doing now, because they see the situation from a different paradigm.

Influences on Sexual Behavior

Teen pregnancy has been associated with poor family support. Though this did not appear to be true in Sara's family, I shared how the pregnancy rate increases among adolescents who lack emotional support from their parents. Single-parent or blended families seem to be especially vulnerable. Up to 80 percent of teen pregnancies occurred in families where the father had left or in which the daughter described her relationship with her stepfather as poor.[15] Young women with serious family difficulties are three times more likely to have had sex with their current boyfriend (usually within two months of establishing the relationship) than women who have a stable family.[16] Perhaps this stems from the emotional need to attach themselves to a male figure. Most girls view their relationships as long-term and plan to spend the rest of their lives with the boyfriend. Therefore, they see sexual expression in this intimate relationship as part of the bonding process.

Sara's friendships were particularly interesting to me because peer relationships influence sexual activity among youth. Teens gather information from each other and incorporate the beliefs into a framework for action. The information may not be accurate. Males often exaggerate their sexual activity to look cool to their friends. This places tremendous pressure on the other young men to conform to an imaginary standard. When teens believe one or two of their close friends have had intercourse, they are six times as likely to initiate the activity. This increases to twenty times when they believe most of their friends have had intercourse.[17] Perceptions of peers may determine a teen's future.

Most girls meet their future boyfriends at places where they hang out during unsupervised time. A survey of youth divided girls into two groups, high-risk and low-risk for pregnancy. The high-risk girls tended to meet boys at parks, bus stops, on public transportation or the street. The young men were often troubled with problem behavior. The boy-girl relationship often resulted in the young woman feeling powerless and giving in to the male's desires.

In comparison, the low-risk women met their future boyfriends at social or recreational clubs, with regular, supervised activities. College brings with it a new social independence, free of tight supervision. College freshmen are particularly at risk for sexual diseases and pregnancy, as they become involved in adult relationships. Parents are not on site to offer advice or restrict actions. The mere presence of parents may deter some actions, just as the sight of a police car reduces speeding on the freeway.

Alcohol and drugs have a direct effect on adolescent sexuality, lowering inhibitions and impairing judgment. Male and female high-school students report increased participation in sexual activity if under the influence of either of these two substances.[18] Fifty-five percent of teens in another survey reported a belief that alcohol and drugs are strongly linked to unintended pregnancy.[19]

Television is the number-one entertainment form in our culture. Sara admitted that she watched TV about six hours a day. Like Sara, most youth spend countless hours absorbing messages from teen sitcoms and advertisements. Sexually explicit programs that depict intimate relationships in soap-opera style fail to reflect the risk and reality of teen parenthood. Sixty-six percent of the public say there is too much sex on TV and that it influences teens sexually, while about 35 percent of teens admit movies and TV encourage them to engage in sexual activity.[20] Sex is seen as an activity that everyone is doing, therefore it must be an expectation. Too many youth never hear a holistic perspective, including the spiritual along with the physical.

A Choice to Make

The current generation has redefined morality. The Bible-based idea of right and wrong at times appears forgotten. Thirty-three percent of teens and adults think premarital sex is a mistake, not because it is morally wrong, but because of the possibility of disease and pregnancy.[21] Most teens do not consider morality as a reason for postponing sexual activity.[22]

I asked Sara about her religious beliefs and if she was affiliated with a church. She affirmed a relationship with Christ. This gave me a Christian base from which to discuss sexuality. We looked at Genesis 2:24, which speaks of a man and woman becoming "one flesh" after marriage. Sara and I then explored the pamphlet *Sex Was Never Meant to Kill You*[23] and followed the outline.

Sara had a choice: to have sex or to save sex for a faithful marriage relationship. The former choice was sullied by the real danger of sexually transmitted disease and the resulting emotional turmoil. Saving sex until marriage focused on taking control of her life. We discussed ways to say *no*. I encouraged her to have a plan before she went on a date, including being selective about whom she would date. She could also select date activities that promote getting to know each other on levels other than the sexual and avoid isolated or sexually stimulating places. Group dating is a healthy option.

We role-played situations that allowed her to respond by saying *no* to the most common "come on" lines. We discussed escape plans for times when she found herself in trouble. I assured Sara that she could start over, that it's never too late. Committing to *secondary virginity* would allow her to take control of her life and live the way Christ intended. The Scriptures are clear that sex outside of marriage is not an option for a

Christian. Sara knew in her heart that this was true, even though it was hard to do the right thing.

The Outcome

It was important for me to discuss initiatives with Sara and her mom that would address spiritual needs, as well as health care needs. Sara had to make a spiritual decision about the sin in her life. Unfortunately, she did not feel she could give up sex at this time and therefore was not willing to repent of an action she planned to continue. She asked if I knew a counselor she could talk to about her moral dilemma. I gave her the name of a youth pastor and assured her of God's love and my continued prayers.

To meet her health needs, Sara needed a physical exam, including tests for sexually transmitted diseases and pregnancy. Preventive counseling consisted of all available methods of contraception and disease prevention, including abstinence. Sara and her mother asked for birth control pills, stating that pregnancy was their biggest concern. I had an ethical decision to make. Should I honor the patient's autonomy and provide what society would consider normal care?

A popular question today is, "What would Jesus do?" Would he provide birth control to prevent the results of an action he had condemned in Scripture? Some Christian providers believe he would, to prevent breaking the relationship by non-acceptance. By maintaining the relationship, Jesus could further influence the young woman's action. Although this sounds reasonable, I cannot find a scriptural basis to support it. I explained that as a Christian provider, I was concerned with the physical and spiritual consequences that may result from their decision. I could not be a part of this plan but would provide the test results necessary for Sara to receive the requested hormones from the county clinic.

Sara's mother was surprised to learn a health care group would not prescribe birth control pills for her daughter, but she accepted the relationship of our beliefs and practice. Although the result was not what I had wished, I prayed for Sara's protection and asked God to strengthen her convictions. I know Sara heard the truth and may recall it at a providential time. This seed may still bear fruit.

Today's youth are confronted with struggles that no generation has faced. Pressures surround every facet of their lives, while they struggle to identify who they are in this world. Their sexual identity is tender and capable of being molded by outside forces. Adults must guard this precious resource and stand prepared to assist throughout the teens' maturation. Knowledgeable nurses are well suited to assist youth and parents with sexual issues, focusing on prevention while providing primary care. We can assist parents in talking openly and honestly with their children. We can be role models of a strong ethic with absolutes the teen can grasp. Together, we can build positive peer pressure to assist our adolescents, save lives and improve the quality of our future leaders.

Originally published in JCN, Summer, 2000

NOTES

1 Cynthia Starr, "Beyond the Birds and the Bees," *Patient Care* 31, no. 7 (April 1997): 103-05.

2 Glenn T. Stanton, *Why Marriage Matters: Reasons to Believe in Marriage in Post-Modern Society* (Colorado Springs: Pinon Press, 1997).

3 Starr, "Beyond the Birds": 103-05.

4 Ibid.; Catherine Burns and others, *Pediatric Primary Care: A Handbook for Nurse Practitioners* (Philadelphia: W. B. Saunders, 1996).

5 Starr "Beyond the Birds": 103-105.

6 Brenda Cobb, "Communication Types and Sexual Protective Practices of College Women," *Public Health Nursing* 14, no. 5 (1997): 293-99.

[7] Ibid.

[8] Carole Morgan, George Chapar and Martin Fisher, "Psychosocial Variables Associated with Teenage Pregnancy," *Adolescence* 30, no. 118 (summer 1995): 277-89.

[9] National Campaign to Prevent Teen Pregnancy, "Nita Lowey and Michael Castle Announce the Formation of a Congressional Advisory Panel" (1998), on-line: http://www.house.gov/lowey/pregnant.htm.

[10] Edward J. Mayeaux Jr. "Pelvic Examination and Vaginal Infections" (1998), on-line: http://lib-sh.lsumc.edu/fammed/compcare/pelvics.html.

[11] Centers for Disease Control and Prevention National Center for HIV, STD and TB Prevention (November 1996), on-line:http://www.cdc.gov/nchstp/dstd/STD_Prevention_in_the_United_States.htm.

[12] Centers for Disease Control and Prevention National Center for HIV, STD and TB Prevention (October 1997), on-line: http://www.cdc.gov/nchstp/dstd/Genital_Herpes_facts.htm.

[13] Arnot Ogden Medical Center, Health on Demand, "Human Papilloma Virus and Genital Warts" (1998), on-line: http://www.aomc.org/copyright.html.

[14] Cleo Rodriquez and Nelwyn Moore, "Perceptions of Pregnant/Parenting Teens: Reframing Issues for an Integrated Approach to Pregnancy Problems," *Adolescence* 30, no. 119 (Fall 1995): 685-705.

[15] Ibid.

[16] Susan Pawlby, Alice Mills and David Quinton, "Vulnerable Adolescent Girls: Opposite-Sex Relationships," *Journal of Child Psychology and Psychiatry and Allied Disciplines* 38, no. 8 (August 1997): 909-20.

[17] Elizabeth Alexander and John Hickner, "First Coitus for Adolescents: Understanding Why and When," *Journal of the American Board of Family Practice* 10, no. 2 (March/April 1997): 96-103.

[18] S. Marie Harvey and Clarence Spigner, "Factors Associated with Sexual Behavior Among Adolescents: A Multivariate Analysis," *Adolescence* 30, no. 118 (summer 1995): 253-63.

[19] National Campaign to Prevent Teen Pregnancy, "What the Polling Data Tell Us: A Summary of Past Surveys on Teen Pregnancy" (1997) on-line: http://www.teenpregnancy.org/Polling.htm.

[20] Ibid.; Starr.

[21] National Campaign, "What the Polling Data Tell Us."

[22] Alexander and Hickner: 96-103.

[23] AAA Women's Services: Why kNOw, "Sex Was Never Meant to Kill You," pamphlet available at: 6232 Vance Road, Chattanooga, TN 37421; (423) 892-0803.

32

Empowering Teens to Say Yes to Abstinence

Kamalini Kumar

For too many years, leaders in our schools, communities, and even churches, have disdained the idea of abstinence-based sex education for our teenagers. The usual answer is always, "It's too unrealistic. Today's teenagers are going to have sex, no matter what. They need birth control, not programs promoting abstinence." As nurses, we have seen first-hand the effects of unwanted pregnancies, abortions and sexually transmitted diseases among our teens, and it becomes easy to buy into the *Band-Aid*™ answer of safe sex and birth control.

But as Christian nurses, we know that God said in his Word a long time ago that illicit sex, though a private act between two individuals, still has potentially widespread, horrendous, physical, social, political, economical, emotional and moral implications. As Josh McDowell says in his book *Why Wait?*: when we break God's loving commandments, the price is awesome. No, sex is not a private act when:

- Unwanted children pay the price
- The public pays the price
- It results in deadly public epidemics

Young people clearly need and want more information, especially on the *why* of sexual relationships rather than the *how*. The so-called sexual revolution has created a dangerous moral precipice from which many youth are falling into destruction. The school-based health clinics and sex education programs have obviously done little or nothing to prevent this.

However, the voice of the culture is being challenged by the teenagers themselves. In talking with some of them, I have learned that they are bucking a system that repeatedly tells them, "All kids are having sex." These young people want to show the world that not all kids are having sex and that they are in control of their passions and not vice-versa.

As a nurse and a Christian, I continued to encourage these adolescents that postponing intercourse until marriage is the best way to ensure loving, satisfying relationships for all of life. Abstinence is not just saying *no,* but it is empowering teens to say *yes* to the right things: building stronger physical and emotional health and protecting their self-esteem and worth in God's eyes. It's about developing character traits of self-control, courage and temperance that will stay with them forever.

I wanted to be involved in the education of these young people, not just in abstinence education, but in Christian character training. I began teaching a series of classes in junior and senior high Sunday school on "Sex Education, God's Curriculum," using Josh McDowell's and Dick Day's book *Why Wait?*

As parents, leaders, teachers and nurses, we need to equip ourselves to address adequately the delicate yet difficult issues of sexuality. We need to provide our young people with down-to-earth answers that make sense to them spiritually, socially, psychologically and physically.

As the Sunday-school lessons progressed, parents heard about them and talked to me about teaching in the school system. I knew this would be a challenging task but began to pray about how I could begin. I agreed to be on the school district's AIDS Education Committee and often found myself the lone dissident voice on issues discussed. This committee evolved into the sex education committee of the school district, where curriculum was designed and created.

I had to learn to be gracious and tactful while consistently insisting that our young people need much more than sex education. They need character trait development in abstinence in all areas of life, including tobacco, drugs, alcohol and gang-related activities, many of which involve sexual activity. Abstinence, I asserted, should be the number one priority in curriculum design. I clearly remember the looks of disdain, ridicule, and even anger, on the faces of some of the committee members, but eventually they produced a document that reflected that priority.

I was then approached by representatives of the Parent-Teacher Associations of the public and Christian schools of a neighboring town, who had heard of my interest. They asked me to teach the program for grades five through eight in their school systems. This was the opening I had been waiting for and, even though it was not in my school district, it gave me the opportunity to reach young people. It is important to gain the support and trust of parents, so I prepared an hour's presentation of the program to be given to parents every year before I begin the program. I developed a program that built on itself from grades five through eight.

Since I taught the same students for four years, it was easy to build rapport with them year after year. I have been doing this for the past eight years. The PTA pays me an honorarium for my time, but the results are worth far more.

I would encourage, no, challenge, all Christian nurses who have a burden for our youth to become involved in this way. We have the knowledge base, respect, credibility and validity of our God-given profession to be used in a mighty way to further extend his kingdom.

Originally published in JCN, Summer, 2000

33

Mobilizing an AIDS Ministry in Your Church

By Lon Solomon

Three years ago, if a nurse or other health care professional had come to me and suggested that our church begin a ministry to AIDS sufferers, I would have been polite, but I would have ignored the suggestion.

When I first heard about AIDS (Acquired Immune Deficiency Syndrome), I didn't pay one bit of attention to it. It seemed like an obscure malady, a problem of homosexuals and drug users.

We didn't have that kind of constituency at McLean Bible Church. Our community is upwardly mobile, high-paced and affluent. We have no slums, tenements, Adonis Clubs, gay bars or heroin alleys. So I dismissed AIDS, believing it really didn't pertain to me or my ministry.

Then, about two years ago, a young man who had grown up in our church called me. "Lon, I have AIDS," he said. "I'm going to die. What am I going to do? You are my pastor—help me!"

Suddenly God had taken AIDS and dropped it right in my lap. I didn't know what to tell this young man. How could I help him? Who in McLean Bible Church was knowledgeable enough to give him the support system that he needed? Even if I could find willing volunteers, where could they get the training for such a ministry?

As a church, we were totally unprepared to help this young man. And I'm convinced that most churches in America are exactly where we were then.

Another Cry for Help

Soon afterward, we had another encounter with AIDS. Our staff member, pastor of evangelism and discipleship, went to get new tires on his car. He took the only vacant seat in the waiting room, right next to a somewhat frail-looking young fellow.

They began to talk, and our staff member soon won the man's confidence. Right there in that sardine-can waiting room, he turned to our staff member and said, "I've got AIDS. I'm dying, and nobody wants anything to do with me anymore. My friends have all forsaken me; my lover's thrown me out; my parents won't talk to me. And you know the worst part of all? It's not that I'm going to die—it's that I'm going to die alone!"

Then the young man hung his head and, in the presence of a half-dozen very uncomfortable onlookers, began to sob. Our staff member put his arm around him, hugged him and said, "Son, I have some really good news for you." Later that week, our staff member introduced him to Jesus Christ.

But the story doesn't end there. The young man wanted to come to church, so our staff member began bringing him. However, we had no support system for him.

Our staff member visited him regularly, but he needed more than that. He needed ordinary, everyday, born-again Christians to rally around him, to hold him up, to understand—at least in part—what he was going through, and to shower him with the love of Jesus. But we didn't have such people.

The young man left us after a few months, saying that he was going to the Midwest to meet some friends. Instead he went to a motel, paid in advance for two days, hung a "Do not disturb" sign on his door and swallowed handfuls of pills. The maid found him two days later, lying dead in his own vomit.

You might ask, "Do you feel responsible for his suicide?" Not ultimately, but partially. As a church, we simply did not have the support system that he needed and that others like him so desperately need.

Much that I have said won't surprise you nurses. As you see more and more AIDS cases, the human drama is becoming all too familiar.

You understand the loneliness and the agony of rejection that people with AIDS suffer. You see how open they are to the gospel. You appreciate the enormous mission field God has laid at the church's door. And most of you probably realize how woefully inadequate most churches' responses have been so far.

So what can you do? How can you help mobilize your church to get involved in reaping a harvest for Jesus among these desperate and needy people?

As I have already said, if some nurses had come to me asking questions like these two years ago, I would have flat ignored them. I would have agreed with them intellectually, but I already had more plates to spin than I could handle. I wouldn't have been excited about trying to spin another one, especially one that seemed irrelevant for the needs of our church.

But, after direct experience with people who had AIDS, I was convinced; I knew God wanted us to develop an AIDS ministry at McLean Bible Church. I began to prepare the way by preaching and teaching about Jesus' compassion and forgiveness.

Now we have nearly forty people involved in some way with HIV-positive people. Some minister to the homeless, compassionately aware of those who also have the AIDS virus. Others pick up people with AIDS who want to attend church and bring them to the services on Sunday morning. Several parishioners have befriended these AIDS sufferers and give them more extensive support.

Some from our congregation visit people with AIDS in hospitals. These lay people received training from Love & Action, a Christian AIDS ministry in Annapolis, Maryland. The same organization coordinates their visits to local hospitals.

You may ask your pastors to start an AIDS ministry. But don't be surprised if they initially ignore your suggestion.

Still, if your goal is to mobilize churches to get involved in AIDS ministry, pastors are the key. They must pick up the passion and sense the burden in their own souls.

In most churches, this will only happen when God shoves the pastors into the kind of situations that he shoved me into. It will probably take people in the churches getting AIDS and dying before the pastors become sensitized to the issues. This process will occur in God's timing and providence; it is out of your control.

Preparing the Way

Does this mean that nurses with a burden for ministry to people with AIDS should do nothing until pastors suddenly catch the vision? Absolutely not! Here are some practical suggestions for what you can do in the meantime:

1) Get prepared for the day when your church is ready to mobilize for an AIDS ministry. Several organizations are helping people with AIDS. Read their literature, and listen to their tapes. If a parachurch organization near you is reaching out to AIDS sufferers, get involved with it so you can receive training in practical ministry skills.

2) Ask your pastor for permission to start and lead a group of volunteers in the church who want to learn about ministering to people with AIDS. Ask to have bulletin announcements or a bulletin-board display. This small band of trained laypeople can form the nucleus of an AIDS ministry when your church as a whole is ready for it.

3) Begin actively praying. Ask God to show the people and leadership of your church the enormous mission field that exists among AIDS patients.

Prejudice is one of the greatest obstacles to AIDS ministry in local churches. Many Christians believe that AIDS is a homosexual disease, a judgment from God on dirty, depraved sinners who deserve whatever they get. No church can begin an AIDS ministry until this kind of unbiblical prejudice is wiped away. Our job as Christians is not to pass judgment on how people got AIDS but to reach out to them with the love, compassion and forgiveness of Jesus Christ.

Many pastors and churches need a heart change before they will be ready for a ministry change. Only God can transform hearts on tough issues like these; he will, in response to your persevering prayer.

God has laid before us an enormous mission field—and it's only going to get bigger. The church has a tremendous opportunity: we can show the world that the same Jesus who befriended publicans and prostitutes in the first century is the friend of homosexuals, drug addicts and AIDS patients in the 20th century.

These people are incredibly open to the gospel. In the Washington, DC area, over 75 percent of the AIDS patients we visit give their lives to Jesus Christ. This is a staggering figure, but it shouldn't shock us. After all, Jesus told us that it is the sick who need the Great Physician and are most receptive to him.

The fields are white unto harvest, not just with lost humanity but with AIDS sufferers. Thank God for nurses who have the passion and courage to reach out to them with the love of Jesus. May God bless and guide you as you challenge your churches to obey God in ministering to people with AIDS.

Originally published in JCN, Summer, 1989

34

Keeping People Healthy
Parish Nursing's Role in Continuous Quality Improvement

Patti Ludwig-Beymer, Cindy M. Welsh & Wendy Tuzik Micek

The term *health care* is often used to describe *sickness care,* referring to services provided by physicians, nurses and other personnel in hospitals or other medical settings. As this type of care has become increasingly technical, churches have tended to view themselves as outside of the health care system.

However, the concept of *holistic health care* has shifted to include health promotion and wellness activities, provided in the home, church, school, workplace and community. Churches are becoming aware of their role in keeping people healthy and are viewing themselves as essential links in health care.

Churches want to contribute to healthier communities.[1] In fact, studies have linked churches and spirituality to better control of hypertension, healthier behaviors in college students, lower suicide rates, diminished pain in patients with cancer and fewer psychological disorders when encountering similar levels of stress.[2]

The concept of holistic health care allows congregations to promote health, not medicine or treatment. One way churches have opted to make this contribution is through the parish nurse ministry.

According to Granger Westberg, the parish nurse serves as: (1) health educator; (2) personal health counselor; (3) coordinator of volunteers; (4) referral source; and (5) integrator of faith and health.[3] A parish nurse has ample opportunity to view both holistic and medical care and bridges these two worlds, speaking both languages and helping the parishioner to negotiate the medical system while preserving holism.

While the United States has a reputation for excellence in medical or sickness care, it is in the midst of a health care crisis. Driven by concerns about cost and access, the health care industry is questioning the quality and appropriateness of care. Throughout health care, we hear of *total quality management* and *continuous quality improvement*. As a provider of community-based services, the parish nurse is in an ideal position to improve the quality of health care offered to individuals, families and communities.

Continuous quality improvement (CQI) has been embraced by health care in an effort to improve processes and better serve the needs of clients. God recognized man's need for advice in order to continually improve: "Better is a poor but wise youth than an old but foolish king, who will no longer take advice" (Eccles 4:13). Continuous quality improvement requires a systematic methodology, known as the scientific method or problem solving model. This model guides quality improvement efforts

Table 1. Process Improvement Models

Scientific Method	Six-Step Process Improvement Model	Focus—PDSA	Eight-Step Process Improvement Model	PRIDE	FADE	Joiner
Observe.	1. Identify and select a problem.	F = **Find** a process to improve. O = **Organize** individuals who know the process.	1. **Focus**—Select and define an opportunity. Determine the magnitude of the opportunity. Assign responsibilities to study the opportunity.	Choose a **process** to improve.	**Focus** on a problem.	Understand the process. Describe the process.
	2. Analyze the problem causes.	C = **Clarify** current knowledge of the process. U = **Understand** the causes of process variation.	2. **Examine**—Understand the current process. Identify customer-supplier relationships. Estimate the cost of poor quality. Determine desired objectives.	Collect data on **relevant** dimensions of performance.	**Analyze** it.	Identify customer needs and concerns.
General Hypothesis.	3. Generate potential solutions.	S = **Select** a strategy for improvement.	3. **Diagnose**—Analyze root causes of process breakdown.	**Interpret** data and evaluate variance.		
Design Plans.	4. Select and plan a solution.	P = **Plan** the improvement and the data collection.	4. **Prescribe**—Develop a solution. 5. **Prognose**—Select indicators. Develop baseline measures and goals. Determine data collection methods.	**Design** or redesign the process.	**Develop** a plan	Develop a standard process. Eliminate errors Remove slack. Reduce variation.
Implement Plans.	5. Implement solution.	D = **Do** the improvement and the data collection.	6. **Treat**—Manage the implementation. Collect feedback information.	**Execute** the improvement plan.	**Execute** it.	Plan for continuous improvement. (PDCA)
Continue Cycle of Observe, Generate Hypothesis, Design Plan and Implement Plan.	6. Evaluate solution.	S = **Study** or check the results. A = **Act** based on results and lessons learned.	7. **Monitor**—Analyze variation. Monitor impact. 8. **Focus**—Determine areas of further improvements.	Validate improvement by remeasuring.		

Adapted from Keill & Johnson (1994)

Table 2. Process Improvement Steps and Tasks

Process Improvement Steps	Tasks
1. Identifying and selecting problem	• Write problem statement. •Prioritize. •Appoint project team.
2. Analyzing problem causes	•Analyze symptoms and causes. •Collect data. •Analyze cause and effect. •Brainstorm. •Prioritize.
3. Generating potential solutions	•Brainstorm. •Analyze potential helps and hindrance. •Build on each other's ideas.
4. Selecting and planning solution	•Prioritize solutions. •Compare resources and costs. •Clarify tasks/action plan. •Present proposals.
5. Implementing solution	•Control project. •Maintain commitment. •Plan contingencies.
6. Evaluating solution	•Monitor results. •Continue process if necessary.

and provides a common frame of reference for the improvement team. Specific features of the model include a focus on internal and external customers, involvement of the process owners, and measurement and monitoring of the degree of improvement. The goal of problem solving is to achieve a breakthrough in performance.[4]

Figure 1. Parish Nursing as Central to Process Improvement

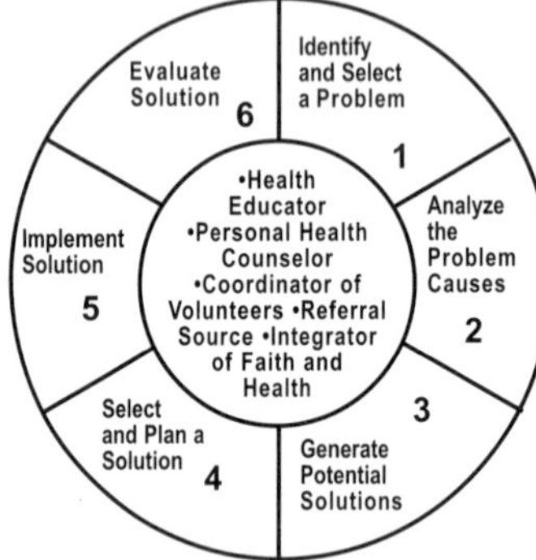

Organizations have proposed and are using many models. Most of them have a common philosophy, although the words and the steps vary slightly depending on the emphasis of style.[5] Six different CQI models are shown in Table 1 (page 297).[6]

The core steps in the structure for effective problem solving are:

(1) Identify and select a problem
(2) Analyze the problem causes
(3) Generate potential solutions
(4) Select and plan a solution
(5) Implement a solution and
(6) Evaluate the solution.

Each step involves a series of tasks. These tasks are described in table two (page 298).[7]

Parish nurses may become involved in all the steps of continuous quality improvement (figure 1, page 298). Six potential activities for parish nurses are:

(1) Identify clinical processes in need of improvement
(2) Participate on multi-disciplinary teams to design clinical improvement products
(3) Plan and implement clinical improvement programs
(4) Develop and use patient education materials
(5) Evaluate the effectiveness of clinical improvement efforts
(6) Revise the products as necessary.

Identify Processes That Need Improvement

By working with the parish population, the nurse is in a unique position to identify opportunities specific to that location. By interacting with the church members, the nurse is able to evaluate the prevalence of various disease processes. Once a specific disease is targeted, the parish nurse may participate on a clinical quality improvement team that will benefit her parish through program development. With a community-based practice, a parish nurse contributes the knowledge of what it takes to support individuals in the home so that institutionalization can be avoided whenever possible.

Help Design Clinical Improvement Products

Since the literature supports the use of clinical improvement products such as pathways, algorithms and guidelines, participating on teams to design these tools will enhance the parish nurse's knowledge of the specific disease and the ability to help clients and families better manage the condition. Parish nurses provide a community health, holistic perspective that combines physical, mental and spiritual components. They are able to sensitize a multidisciplinary team to a client's spiritual needs in times of illness or in making a long-term health or lifestyle adjustment. Therefore, parish nurse participation on these teams offers the opportunity to assure user-friendly products appropriate for the congregation.

Implement Clinical Improvement Programs

Through their community-based work, parish nurses have a population in which to utilize continuum programs that the traditional hospital-based nurse may lack. The ambulatory population's needs are as unique as those of the hospitalized patient. In planning and developing clinical improvement programs, the parish nurse can assure that the interests of clients in the congregation are considered and encompassed in the program.

For example, support groups are an essential part of chronic disease management. The parish nurse has a responsibility to integrate spiritual aspects into the support group to address the needs of the members holistically. Incorporating spiritual support allows the parish nurse to identify and resolve issues that would not have surfaced otherwise. Prayer may also be a powerful adjunct to clinical care and modifications of lifestyle related to the management of chronic illness.

Use Patient Education Materials

Patient-friendly tools, written in educationally appropriate language, need to be identified or developed and then utilized. These tools can greatly assist the parish nurse in educating clients on specific disease processes. They may also reinforce the verbal education provided by parish nurses in individual and group encounters. Although the patient's needs are always at the heart of product development, usefulness cannot be determined until the tools are actually put into use. Parish nurses are aware of church members' demographics and educational and spiritual needs, and can work to assure these are addressed in the development of educational materials. Their efficacy can be tested through use with appropriate clients in the congregation.

Evaluate Clinical Improvement Efforts

The parish nurse is in a wonderful position to test the products developed by the clinical CQI team and needs to be part of the measurement plan to identify what measures are most meaningful to the congregation. Through expertise in measuring outcomes, necessary for evaluating the effectiveness of any clinical improvement effort, the parish nurse can provide valuable community-based data that encompass the holistic, spiritual approach to providing health care.

Revise As Necessary

With a community-based, congregation-specific practice, who could better test the process of an improvement effort than the parish nurse? Products are used in the field on a daily basis. The feedback the parish nurse can provide on the products and the implementation process is invaluable in guiding the need for further revisions and/or enhancements, as well as for future efforts in the area of clinical quality improvement.

An Example

Marge is a parish nurse in a low-income, inner-city congregation. She notices that parishioners of all ages come to her with respiratory problems, often saying they have a "touch of asthma." Marge tries to keep up with the current literature but finds it hard to apply the national guidelines for asthma care in her setting. She sees parishioners who are caught in the cycle of repeated hospitalizations and emergency department visits and knows that care can be improved.

Marge contacts the director of nursing (DON) at a nearby hospital to discuss her concerns. She learns that the hospital is trying to improve their care of individuals with asthma not only within the hospital but also in the community. The hospital realizes that patient education needs to be reinforced at frequent intervals in many settings. The DON asks Marge if she will serve on a CQI team composed of individuals from medicine, nursing, pharmacy and respiratory care. Marge is interested and discusses the opportunity with the pastor of her church, sharing her records and the stories of the parishioners she has seen. The pastor wholeheartedly supports Marge's participation on the team.

When the CQI team convenes, Marge shares appropriate information about her parishioners. Team members see Marge as a valuable team member, with her community perspective and her capacity to view individuals when they are healthy, acutely ill and anywhere in between. Marge reminds the team that a person with asthma not only needs treatment for lungs but has holistic needs as well. She encourages them to look at the context of care, including environment, family support, emotional status and spiritual support.

Marge advocates a continuum-of-care approach to asthma management. The team agrees that the overall goal is to manage individuals outside the hospital setting. Team physicians agree to change the way they prescribe medications and structure the education they provide. In addition, the team incorporates the role of the parish nurse into their program: (1) The parish nurse will continue to counsel individuals and may also refer them to team members if further education or therapy is needed; (2) The parish nurse will host a series of group sessions on asthma management, with the parish nurse coordinating the sessions and various team members serving as guest speakers; and (3) In collaboration with other community agencies, Marge will assist parishioners in setting up an asthma support group, with sessions beginning with prayer and reflection led by the members. Using her skills, Marge will be attuned to any underlying issues that need to be addressed. The team reviews and modifies educational materials; Marge recommends that they be kept simple. In response, the team is able to compile material with a fifth-grade reading level. Along with other clinicians, Marge volunteers to try the educational materials with some of her parishioners. Revisions are made to the materials based on their feedback, and the program is implemented.

When the team discusses how they will measure the asthma program's effectiveness, Marge encourages them to look beyond physiological factors to see how individuals are coping with their condition. She helps the team locate an excellent functional status questionnaire that can be administered to individuals in a variety of settings. She advises the team to measure not only days of school or work lost because of asthma symptoms but also important events, such as church services missed by individuals. The team agrees on a measurement plan, and Marge is instrumental in collecting data. Parishioners trust her and are willing to complete the questionnaires because of Marge's involvement.

Is this an actual case study? No, not yet. But the example illustrates the importance of including the parish nurse perspective on clinical improvement teams. It also highlights the many skills brought to the table by the parish nurse. Finally, it demonstrates the importance of a team in changing a care process. No one alone could have the impact achieved by the overall program designed by the multidisciplinary team.

As this example reinforces, parish nurses are in an ideal position to contribute to projects that improve the quality of health care offered to individuals, families and communities. For health care to be holistic and comprehensive, it must include health promotion and wellness activities provided in a variety of community settings. Churches are in a prime position to contribute to healthier communities and improved health care delivery. Parish nurses can lead the way.

Originally published in JCN, Winter, 1998

NOTES

1 L. James Wylie, "The Mission of Health and the Congregation," in Phyllis Solari-Twadell, Anne Marie Djupe & Mary Ann McDermott, eds., *Parish Nursing: The Developing Practice* (Park Ridge, Ill.: National Parish Nurse Resource Center, 1990), p. 25.

[2] David Larson, "Making the Case for Religion in Clinical Care: A Look Back" in *Spiritual Care Research: What We Are Learning* (paper delivered at Mayo Medical Center Conference, Rochester, Minn., November 8, 1996).

[3] Granger Westberg, "A Historical Perspective: Holistic Health and the Parish Nurse," in Phyllis Solari-Twadell, Anne Marie Djupe and Mary Ann McDermott, eds., *Parish Nursing: The Developing Practice* (Park Ridge, Ill.: National Parish Nurse Resource Center, 1990), p. 33.

[4] Paul E. Plsek & Arturo Onnias, *Quality Improvement Tools: Problem Solving Glossary* (Wilton, Conn.: Juran Institute, 1989), p. 1.

[5] Mara M. Melum and Marie Kuchuris Sinioris, *Total Quality Management: The Health Care Pioneers* (Chicago: American Hospital Publishing, 1992), pp. 3-269.

[6] Patricia Keill and Trudy Johnson, "Optimizing Performance Through Process Improvement," *Journal of Nursing Care Quality* 9, no. 1 (1994): 1-9.

[7] John Bank, *The Essence of Quality* (New York: Prentice Hall, 1992), p. 174.

Part Seven

Ideas That Work

35

Health Screening
Pastor at Risk

Susan L. Neff

For the past three years I have conducted monthly health seminars followed by blood pressure checks at First Baptist Church. Since the average age in this faith community is over sixty-five, I considered it important to schedule a talk on strokes. One of our community medical facilities was giving stroke awareness presentations and offering stroke evaluations. I was able to obtain one of the program coordinators to speak to the group, and her talk was well received. She extended an invitation to all those present to take advantage of the free stroke evaluation being offered at the medical facility.

Reverend Lind, the pastor of the church, was enthusiastic that this service was offered to his parishioners. He wanted to be evaluated himself, an encouragement to others to follow his example. Although not a top priority in his busy schedule and in spite of the fact that he exhibited no symptoms, he called and made an evaluation appointment.

A week later I received a call from Pastor Lind, who told me that during his evaluation it was discovered that he had atrial fibrillation, a decided risk factor for strokes. He was immediately scheduled for further testing. As a result of the findings, lifestyle changes were strongly recommended. He was placed on appropriate medication, began an exercise program and made dietary changes that resulted in a thirty-pound weight loss. His energy level has increased and, in general, he feels better than he has for a long time.

Pastor Lind told me that if it had not been for the parish nurse program and the seminars I facilitate, this potentially serious condition with its possible fatal consequences would not have been diagnosed. He now uses his experience as a testimony to the benefits of having a parish nurse associated with the church.

Originally published in JCN, Winter, 1997

36

Toning the Temple
A Church-Based Health Fair

Pamela Stuchlak

I had just finished my Family Nurse Practitioner program and was all fired up to use my new health promotion skills. Besides starting a hospital-based practitioner position, I wanted to spread the *good news* of health promotion in the community. How about starting with my own church? I thought the idea sounded great and took off with it.

Health promotion and disease prevention will be the focus of health care in the future. With skyrocketing medical and hospitalization costs, we cannot afford to be ill. Company profits are eaten away by employee health-insurance claims. People are beginning to understand that by choosing a healthy lifestyle, they are able to control some of the risk factors leading to disease.

James 2:26 says that " . . . faith without works is dead." This sometimes comes to mind when I see patients' families praying for help when the patients smoked all their lives, were very overweight and non-compliant with prescribed care. I Corinthians 6:19

refers to our bodies as temples. Would individuals take better care of themselves if they thought of their bodies and selves as special temples? Combining biblical concepts and health habits may be just what a congregation needs to be motivated to practice healthier lifestyles.

I spoke to other health professionals in the church about spreading the health promotion idea through a health fair. They liked the idea and decided the fair would be called "Toning the Temple."

Interested health professionals met as a group and brainstormed about the focus of the fair. Should it center on seniors, children, heart health, accidents or something else? After looking at the State Department of Health morbidity statistics for the cities where our congregation is located, we decided to focus on prevention of the four leading causes of death in the area: heart disease, cancer, strokes and accidents. By gearing our fair to local needs, it became unique to our congregation. Other fairs I attended did not have such a focus. Some fairs had more of an underlying advertising theme versus a purely health-awareness focus.

The Committee Was On Its Own

Initially, the church board supported the fair but later expressed concern about liability. So the committee was on its own. We sponsored the event ourselves, while still using the church hall facilities. After a successful first experience, the church happily sponsored the fair the following year.

Health Fair Committee members were each given a topic and asked to design or coordinate a booth around the topic. We found many organizations eager to participate, including the American Heart Association, the American Cancer Society, the American Diabetic Association, the American Dairy Association, Emergency Medical Systems, local hospitals, fitness centers, centers for aging, local grocers and other health professionals. Most individuals donated their services or asked permission to advertise; a few asked for a small fee. We raised funds for expenses through a raffle and a donation box at the fair.

These are some of the activities at our health fairs: an RN massage therapist demonstrated a back massage for relaxation; a nutritionist shared recipes and samples of low-fat desserts; a fun one-mile walk; blood pressure screening; Resusci-Annie with basic CPR instruction; glucose checks, a pharmacist gave a talk on blood pressure medications; a dietitian explained how to calculate a 30 percent fat diet; a guest appearance by the "Couch Potato"; low-impact aerobic exercise demonstration, with group participation; a low-fat meal, using the four basic food groups; cancer-screening models of abnormal lumps; pulmonary function screening.

The fair committee was enthusiastic about the fair and wanted as many people as possible to attend. Because space in the hall was limited, we advertised mostly within the congregation but also informed other local churches. Our church included notices about the fair in the congregational newsletter sent out one month before the fair. We announced the fair during the worship service for two Sundays prior to the event and posted fliers throughout the church.

Since the fair was held immediately following the 11 a.m. service, we had a captive audience. The refreshments provided at the fair enticed others into the church hall.

Success Is Sweet

The fair was a success! About seventy-five people attended. Hearing people ask questions, seeing them swap their low-fat recipes and listening to them talk about exercise experiences was rewarding. I was even more excited a few weeks later when I saw several members start walking routines. The fair was a lot of work, but it was worth it.

I'm hoping these fairs will encourage the church and individuals to make health their *policy*. I'll know that's happening when I see low-fat refreshments being served at meetings, when church meals are low in fat and contain the four food groups, when the church sponsors more events that involve exercise, and when the no-smoking rules are enforced for all groups using the building.

"Toning the Temple" was a valuable experience and great fun. As nurses we define our area of practice to be health assessment and maintenance. A church health fair enables us to actively use our skills in the community to promote health. We can make a difference by making things happen. Maybe you could organize a health fair in your church and inspire others to a healthier lifestyle.

Originally published in JCN, Summer, 1992

37

Church Health Fairs
Partying with a Purpose

Pattie Boyes

Mary shares how God is helping her cope with her cancer. Geoff recounts his AIDS story to our church. Carrie describes a twelve-step program for codependency that she leads. John's exhibit features books on health and healing from a Christian bookstore. Joyce, a Christian counselor, discusses sexuality with teens. James offers a whole-person health inventory. In a quiet place, Martha leads meditations that she designed. Joe explains his role of spiritual director at a nearby retreat center.

Encouraging positive choices is basic to health fairs. Life is more than our visible physical bodies. Our thoughts, emotions, personalities and our ability to relate with God, the supernatural and the transcendent are vital to us.[1] For easy identification, we use labels such as body, mind (intellect and emotion) and spirit, but we know that what affects one part of us affects the rest. Long ago King Solomon recorded his observation of this interconnectedness of people, "A cheerful heart is a good medicine, but a downcast spirit dries up the bones" (Prov 17:22).

Although cancer is a physical disease, it impacts people, family members and friends emotionally, spiritually, psychologically, socially, financially and more. Perfect wholeness (health, well-being) is not a destination that we reach in this life. Though we experience setbacks along the way (that is, arthritis, abuse or lack of forgiveness), we journey toward wholeness by our physical, mental and spiritual lifestyle choices. Our body, mind and spirit need to be nourished, exercised and rested.

Health fairs encourage well-being in a festive atmosphere. Exhibits, demonstrations, activities, speakers, one-on-one discussions, mini exercise classes, nutritious food samples, puppet shows and health screening can help people of a church and its surrounding community to make positive lifestyle choices in all aspects of their lives. My challenge was to organize a health fair that would assist in people's journeys toward wholeness. All that I read about, heard about and observed at health fairs encouraged physical (and occasionally mental) health, but before planning our first health fair, I had not found one example of encouraging spiritual health at a health fair.

The two health fairs that I facilitated were a year apart in two parish nurse practices: the first at my own church, the second at another. In each church, I worked with small groups of people who formed a health committee. Throughout our assessment, planning, implementation and evaluation, we prayed for God's guidance and creative ideas. After our fairs, I talked with other parish nurses to learn of their health fair experiences and am including their ideas.

Assessment and Planning

We began by asking, "Who will benefit from a health fair?" We chose the fairs as a means of accomplishing a great deal of health education in one time and place. Our first health fair targeted senior adults. Following that one, a health committee member suggested that we plan a fair for children in the fall, one for women in the winter and a second one for seniors the following spring. That seemed like a good plan for us, although one a year is frequent enough for most organizations.

Our second fair focused on the whole family. Most of the exhibits attracted adults, although children and teens enjoyed some displays. At both health fairs, we included two or more fifteen- to twenty-minute classes. At the second, we planned at least two classes for each age group, with the teens pre-approving the topics for their classes.

Good record keeping (with a database and a camera) at our first health fair helped in planning the second. Other parish nurses agreed. Joanne Kinoshita calls record keeping a template for their next health fair. Photos serve the dual purpose of documentation and promotion. Some committees display photos on their church bulletin boards to report on their health fairs to their congregations.

Next we queried, "Who will help?" We asked people of the church, people they knew and agencies in the community to be involved. People helped us organize, advertise, prepare, exhibit, speak, screen, pick up, set up, buy, prepare and serve food, greet people, take pictures, clean up, return equipment and thank people. We wrote eighty thank-you notes after our second fair. Responding to a need, people of Carol Woodyard's church included a babysitting service for the visitors and volunteers at their women's health fair.

We had many choices to make in our planning. We asked, "When will people come?" We considered Sunday and the regular time that our seniors meet (two Thursday afternoons a month) but decided on Saturday afternoon for both health fairs. We chose 1:00 to 3:00 p.m. This proved good for both groups. The partnership of Lisa Zerull's and Helen Zebarth's churches helped them choose Sunday, 8:30 a.m. to 1:00 p.m., for their health fairs. This suits the dismissal times of each church's two morning services. (They alternate their health fair between the churches annually.) The health fair at Lynette Lannsom's church accommodates their Saturday evening and Sunday morning services.

We looked at each church building and chose to use most of the education, fellowship and kitchen space for exhibits, demonstrations, speakers, videos, food. We used the parish nurse offices for hearing testing. A map served a useful purpose for visitors and exhibitors at Lynette's church because their health fair occupied three separate areas.

We linked both of our health fair themes with the season: Walk into Spring and A Spring Check-up. We used spring flowers (daffodils one year and tulips the next) in the advertising, decorating, programs and thank-you notes.

Food at health fairs should model healthy nutrition and may encourage people to come. We chose fruit and vegetable platters and low-fat muffins. Becky Elbert arranged a fundraiser for a group to sell submarine sandwiches and fruit juices at their all-day health fair. Wonderful baking smells wafting into the sanctuary at Helen's and Lisa's churches helped entice people to come to the health fair after morning worship. Cooking demonstrations and sampling can teach tasty nutrition.

To help pay for our health fairs, we placed a basket by the food for donations. Besides paying for the food, contributions also helped pay for advertising, program folders, reusable nametags, balloons and flowers. Funds designated for parish nursing paid the balance. We also sold Christian books on health and healing.

To keep their health fair from becoming commercial rather than educational, Carol's health committee decided not to sell anything except Christian books related to topics featured at their fair. Some churches pay expenses from a budget, while others welcome a raffle. However, churches that view raffles as gambling do not permit them.

Ethics and common sense require respecting the church's values and standards. At Margo Truett's Catholic church, a natural family planning practitioner was a good fit. I blundered when I booked a water cooler for a Salvation Army community church from a business that also sells beer- and wine-making supplies. I returned to the retailer, explained and booked a water cooler from another source.

We searched for active exhibits and short classes. We had a physically fit young man of the church lead an exercise class. Another qualified man of the church taught basic neck massage. A physiotherapist checked people's balance at a health fair at Margo's church. Anatomical models for practice of breast and testicle self-examination facilitate active learning. Review of cardiopulmonary resuscitation would offer an active learning option.

The visit of a police car was our kids' favorite activity. Other popular activities for kids include bicycle safety and visits by a fire truck and ambulance. For mental activity we utilized a quiz after a safety video, as well as questionnaires concerning hearing, fitness, nutrition and lifestyle. Jane Wilkes's church offered spiritual activity in a meditation room at their women's health day.

We encouraged interaction at all exhibits. We initiated conversation about numbers and their meaning for blood pressure, blood sugar, blood cholesterol, glaucoma, lung function, hearing and body mass index (BMI). People signed consents for invasive procedures. We wished that we had requested permission for follow-up phone calls about abnormal results.

Though we displayed Ask a Nurse, more questions came at individual screening stations. The label Ask a Pharmacist may have given one of our displays more interaction. The Ask a Doc area included doctors, dentists and veterinarians of Lisa's and Helen's churches. Although we allowed a few organizations to send exhibits without a person for interaction, those exhibits received almost no attention.

We found many resources for physical health promotion and some for mental health promotion but had to be innovative in our search for resources to encourage spiritual health. We advertised supportive activities of the church, which could include healing services, support groups, twelve-step groups, classes that combine physical and spiritual exercise, small groups, pastoral care groups, Stephen Ministries and deliverance ministries. We offered a whole-person health check up to encourage people to care for themselves. A counselor and a chaplain were present as spiritual health providers. We presented printed resources from a Christian bookstore and the *Focus on the Family* organization.

At our first health fair, we included results of a survey about how people of our church care for their mental health. Answers encompassed activities that addressed care of body, mind and spirit. The benefits of walking, reading and praying are not specific to just one aspect of our lives. One poster featured spiritual disciplines: meditation, prayer, fasting, worship and others. Scripture posters are an appropriate choice.

Carol noted that a Christian counselor and other individuals from her church were comfortable speaking of their faith in relation to their topics. Helen and Lisa's parish nurse booth included material about how to pray with people. Helen took spiritual care a step further on the day of the health fair by speaking in both morning services about the scriptural basis of whole-person health and parish nursing. Other nurses suggest that spiritual directors, retreat centers and hospice and palliative care groups could be invited to exhibit.

After these choices and planning, we had to encourage people to come. We advertised our health fairs with posters at our church, at neighborhood churches and in the community at businesses, community clubs, libraries and members' apartment buildings. At church we put notices in the bulletin and made announcements from the pulpit. We publicized our health fairs in community newspapers. We encouraged our people to invite friends to come to a non-threatening activity at church. Contacting radio, television and newspapers for interviews could be useful.

Implementation

The evening before the health fairs, we set up tables, chairs, signs and some equipment. On the day of the fair, I tried to take a deep breath, relax and enjoy it. I kept myself free to welcome exhibitors, interact with people and handle whatever happened. For us, "whatever" included exhibitors that unexpectedly did or did not come, a temporarily-missing display and a speaker without an audience.

Evaluation

To help us evaluate our health fairs, we asked our exhibitors and speakers for their written comments and suggestions. Most comments were affirming: "It was a very positive networking experience." "I learned some interesting program concepts." They also remarked on the variety of choices that supported the theme of a health check-up. Balancing those comments, they suggested that we try for a larger space with combined congregations, "Call the local media for more publicity," and change the time of year because: "There are a lot of health shows/ expos during this time frame."

Unwritten evaluation included the enthusiasm of one exhibitor, who asked for help to organize a health fair for his congregation. Informal evaluation showed that we had crowded our exhibitors—they needed more table space and an area to stand without blocking their display. Since part of an evaluation is planning for the next event, we wrote recommendations after each health fair. Thus, for the second fair we made nametags for volunteers before the fair day. We also suggested making a list of photos for a volunteer to take. However, we all forgot cameras at our second health fair.

Asking visitors to evaluate health fairs is common. However, we accepted the recommendation of one health committee member who was strongly against the idea for our group. Emma Begg asked visitors for their general impression of the information, its presentation, how people heard about the health fair, their favorite exhibit and their intended action because of the health fair.[2] This gave the organizers useful information.

A longer-term evaluation question asks, "What impact did the health fair have?" Have people started walking routines? Do they bring healthier foods to meetings and meals? Do they ask more health questions? Shirley has observed lower-fat foods and more variety within the food groups being brought for meals. She is pleased with this progress.

Some things we planned worked, and some did not work in our attempts to assist people on their journeys toward wholeness through health fairs. We gave special attention to active and interactive learning that included lifestyle choices for the well-being of body, mind and spirit. Health fairs provide a fun-filled, high-intensity opportunity to communicate good information about wellness to a church community.

Originally published in JCN, Summer, 2001

NOTES

1 Elizabeth A. Peterson, "Wholeness: Transcending Time and Change," *Journal of Christian Nursing* 15, no. 3 (Summer 1998): 4-9.

2 Emma Begg, "Planning a Health Fair," *Community Outlook* (October 1989): 19-22.

38

Healing Service
An Unexpected Healing

Jean Wright-Elson

Recently my church instituted a service of healing, an accepted but forgotten ritual in the Methodist tradition. In this service, worshipers are invited to come forward and express their concerns to the minister or parish nurse. They are then anointed with consecrated oil using the words, "I anoint you with this oil in the name of the Father, the Son and the Holy Spirit." Although this service is relatively new in my church, it has been enthusiastically embraced by the congregation. As the parish nurse, I especially appreciate the opportunity to participate and to hear the various problems with which people are struggling.

It was in such a service that a tall, slender woman approached me, one in a long line of many waiting to be anointed. She stepped forward and in a soft, breathy voice said, "I wish to be healed of my breast lump." Because of the number of people who come forward, we usually do not have time to respond in depth to the petitions we hear, but the nurse in me had to follow up on this. I leaned forward and whispered in her ear, "I hope you are under treatment."

Her reply jolted me. "No, this is it."

Dear Lord, I thought. *This woman believes my making the sign of the cross on her forehead with oil is going to magically make that lump disappear.* I quickly requested she come to see me which, thankfully, she did.

Jeannette is a fifty-four-year-old divorced woman who noticed the lump eighteen months before seeing me. She had read many articles on faith healing and truly believed that if she prayed and meditated hard enough, God would heal her. She was shy and passive, and easily intimidated by those in the medical profession, especially male physicians.

I listened to Jeannette's fears and concerns, and her deep conviction that miracles can happen with the right kind of prayers. Acknowledging her reluctance to seek medical help, I encouraged Jeannette to think that God imbued physicians with knowledge and skills so they could heal others in Christ's name. It was a long and emotional counseling session, until gradually she saw that her prayers needed to be coupled with appropriate medical intervention. Silently I prayed that Jeannette had not waited too long.

Since finances were limited, she set up an appointment at a low-cost women's clinic. I accompanied her to the clinic, realizing her anxiety level would prevent her from completely understanding what was said. The mammogram revealed that the lump was highly suspicious for malignancy. The physician told her that a biopsy was needed immediately and, in all probability, a radical mastectomy would be necessary. Knowing she needed my continuing care as her parish nurse and fellow church member, I drove her to the hospital for the biopsy. As we progressed through the various procedures and options presented, I continued to guide her with my nursing knowledge and spiritual support.

Throughout this time, I witnessed Jeannette changing from a self-effacing, timid person to one who began to take charge and make decisions for herself. She rejected the clinic physician's proposal for a radical mastectomy, made some inquiries and found an excellent clinic at a highly-rated hospital that was offering breast cancer care to women on limited incomes. Jeannette had a lumpectomy and dissection of nodes, which revealed early stage cancer. She is currently undergoing chemotherapy and radiation.

During this life-changing event, Jeannette has had the support and care of a sister from whom she had previously been emotionally distant. In the process, their relationship has become closer. When bad things happen to us, sometimes good things result. In addition, our weekly prayer group, the ministerial staff and others in the congregation have uplifted Jeannette with their loving prayers of support.

Jeannette did not have the miraculous healing she had ardently prayed for and had to accept medical intervention. However, I believe a miracle did occur. In a letter Jeannette wrote to me she said, "It was divine intervention that I found myself in your line to be anointed rather than the minister's. Although I knew we had a parish nurse, I did not know who you were until I was close enough to read your name tag. At that moment I found the courage to tell why I needed healing."

For me, a relatively new parish nurse, this has been a profound experience. If I have saved one person from a potentially life-threatening illness, then the hard work of developing the health ministry program for my church has been worthwhile. It more than validates the importance of having a nurse as part of the church staff.

Originally published in JCN, Winter, 1997

39

Does God Heal Today?

Marcia L. Denine

Two years ago I attended a healing service conducted by the Order of St. Luke, the Physician (OSL). The OSL is a non-denominational Christian organization dedicated to the practice and preservation of the Christian commission to heal the sick. The commission is carried out through anointing with oil, laying on of hands and prayer.

Since I was a young child, I wondered, *How did Jesus do that?* I recall listening to my grandmother tell the stories of Jesus, walking among the sick and healing the blind, the lame, the dumb and the mute. In parochial school the nuns would tell us about Jesus walking many miles along dusty roads to speak of the glory of God and his kingdom and to touch those who hurt in order to heal them. *How?* I wondered.

As an adult at the OSL healing service, I knew deep within my heart that Jesus healed because he had compassion and mercy on those who suffer. He healed because he loved. He healed because he is God. He gave authority to his followers to do the same. As I went forward to be dedicated as an associate member of the order, I knew Jesus had answered the inquiry of a child, "How did you do that?"

Previously, when I had attended an OSL healing service at the same church, I had been suffering for months from intense neck and shoulder pain. Over-the-counter pain relievers had not eased the discomfort. After being anointed with oil and prayed for, as someone sang "Lord, Don't Take Your Joy from Me," I left the service, still suffering nearly unbearable pain in my neck and shoulders. I prayed and thanked God for the peaceful experience I'd had and for the strength to accept his will for healing, or not healing, my pain. The next morning I awoke with no discomfort. The pain has never returned.

Healing is a part of our Christian heritage. The Gospels record that in Christ's three years of ministry on earth, he spent much of his time healing the sick. Wherever he walked, people gathered, seeking his healing touch. Even the demon-possessed recognized his authority. Toward the end of his ministry, he authorized many to go out and heal the sick in his name. It's this that makes healing our Christian heritage: not so much that Jesus himself healed, but that he authorized many of his followers to do the same.

In the book of James, we are advised to anoint the sick with oil. "Are any among you sick? They should call for the elders of the church and have them pray over them, anointing them with oil in the name of the Lord. The prayer of faith will save the sick, and the Lord will raise them up; and anyone who has committed sins will be forgiven" (Jas 5:14-15).

Christ directed the twelve, "Freely you have received, freely give" (Mt 10:8 NIV). The apostles had walked with, talked with, eaten with, prayed with and lived with the Master. Daily they observed the Creator re-creating. Places demons once inhabited, the Master made clean. Where doubt once festered, the Master made believers. The lame walked. The blind could see. The dead were raised. The apostles saw it all. It was their reality: life in the kingdom of Light. They were instructed to go out and do the same. Surely, the Lord instructed them to do something they were entirely capable of doing, because of him. If they would go out and heal in Christ's name, he would heal.

In the book of Acts, we see the apostles continuing in the work to which Christ Jesus had commissioned them, healing the sick and casting out demons. The practice of Christian healing has been passed down from believer to believer since the first century.

I pray more fervently for my patients now, believing Christ's healing touch will be with them. Recently I prayed for two patients with methicillin-resistant staphylococcus aureus (MRSA). Two wound cultures were sent on each patient, and the results after seventy-two hours were negative for MRSA.

I prayed for a man who had stopped eating and taking his medications. He had declared his desire to die but continued on IVs. He was already bed-bound, too weak to tolerate sitting up in a chair. Eventually, he was barely responsive, only occasionally opening an eye to acknowledge a family member's presence. His respirations were rapid and shallow. His color was pallid. His lungs and ankles began to accumulate fluid, and his urinary output diminished. Death appeared to be imminent. But one day, out of the blue, he asked for Jello.™ Slowly he began taking fluids and food. IVs were discontinued. He asked to get out of bed. He rallied!

Another older gentleman I prayed for was experiencing weakness on his left side, slurred speech, urinary incontinence and confusion. A CT head scan revealed a possible acute infarction in an area where a chronic infarction had been previously diagnosed. After three days of decline, the patient arose early one morning, washed and dressed independently, and ambulated with his walker to the nurses' station to inquire, "How long until breakfast?" All previously noted symptoms have resolved.

These are not people I have deliberately laid hands on with the intention of praying for healing or anointed with oil. These are patients I prayed for in the normal course of my care for them: while doing treatments, checking neuro signs or taking vitals. They are people I prayed for on my way to work or in my early morning devotions. Only the Lord knows the extent of his intervention for each of these patients. Yet, I firmly believe I interceded for these patients before a Lord of mercy, a Lord who heals, a Lord who is God.

"Jesus Christ is the same yesterday and today and forever" (Heb 13:8). He still moves mountains. He still heals the sick, casts out demons and raises the dead to life in the kingdom of Light.

Originally published in JCN, Spring, 2000

40

Documenting Congregational Nursing Care

A Model

Renae Schumann

Congregational or parish nursing care requires documentation as does any other field of nursing. Documentation of client, family or the congregation during each stage of the nursing process is crucial to the delivery of quality care and to the enhancement of the practice.

Congregational nursing care is more likely to be effective when it is well documented from the onset of the nurse's contact with the client. Documentation during each stage of the nursing process leads to efficient and effective care, as well as improved communication among those involved in the care. The more effective the care, the greater the opportunity for the growth and acceptance of congregational nursing within the faith community and nursing profession.

While developing the curriculum for the Congregational Care Nursing and Congregational Nurse Practitioner master's programs at Houston Baptist University, the faculty created a tool suitable for documentation of congregational nursing. This tool, the Holistic Care Summary (page 333), incorporates the five steps of the nursing process and flows from the common parish nursing roles, the principles of holistic nursing care, teaching-learning theory and growth and development theory.

Molly: A Case Study

Molly, an elderly woman, asked the congregational nurse to take her blood pressure, stating that it "just doesn't feel right today." While the nurse took the blood pressure, Molly started to talk about her husband, who had died from a stroke on that same date one year before, and about the loss of sleep she had experienced since her husband's death. She indicated that she was worried about her blood pressure because her husband's had always been high. Molly stated that she didn't want to have the same problems that he had before he died.

Molly said she felt she was responsible for her husband's death because she had not learned about proper dietary control of hypertension until it was too late. She said she was afraid that if other people knew she had "killed" her husband, she would never again be allowed to be part of the congregation. She started to cry, saying that she felt guilty about her husband but that she wanted to get on with her life. She wanted to be with her Christian brothers and sisters but was afraid of their rejection.

The nurse told Molly her blood pressure was 190/105. Through assessment and questioning, the nurse learned that Molly had a strong faith in God but without children to whom to pass on that belief, she felt alone in the world. She had completed the fourth grade but had to quit school after that to help support the family. Molly said that she had always been able to learn by watching people and imitating them. She did not know how to drive and had depended on her husband to take her where she needed to go. Now she had nobody to drive her to the store, to the doctor or even to church.

Molly stated that she felt helpless and wanted her life to end but was afraid that God would never forgive her for the death of her husband, and that she was doomed to spend eternity away from God. She began to cry again, stating that she no longer wanted to live but that she was afraid to die.

The nurse saw many areas of need in which she as the congregational nurse could intervene to promote holistic wellness and thus improve the quality of Molly's life. The Holistic Care Summary was used to begin development of Molly's care plan.

Planning Molly's Care

The nurse completed the personal data section with Molly's name, age and birthdate. Molly had disclosed a prominent life event, the death of her husband a year ago. She stated she had no children and that she felt alone, so the nurse listed no current support systems.

The fact that Molly had only completed the fourth grade would have a major impact on the methods used to deliver her care, so the nurse wrote a detailed entry in the teaching/learning sections. Molly stated that she learned best by observation and imitation, so that was listed under preferred learning style. A barrier to learning included limited reading ability, while a learning strength was her apparent motivation, as indicated by seeking the help of the nurse. Experiences with learning seemed limited to those shared with her late husband.

In completing the Objective-Subjective Holistic Needs Assessment section, the nurse identified numerous physical, emotional and spiritual needs that would require intervention within many of the congregational nurse roles. Molly's physical needs included teaching and counseling regarding effects, management and prevention of the complications of hypertension; referral to her physician and to other agencies for hypertension; advocacy in helping her get to and from the doctor's office, to the store for proper food and to church.

Molly's emotional needs focused on her feelings of being alone and her desire to be back among her Christian brothers and sisters. Her emotional needs overlapped her spiritual needs, in that her aloneness was apparently partially self-imposed out of her fear of rejection. The nurse listed the need to refer Molly to the church's seniors group and to draw advocacy from that group.

Molly had many spiritual needs, serious enough to prevent her healing if improperly managed. She needed teaching and counseling about the love and grace of God and about forgiveness. Molly also needed to deal with her grief and the associated guilt. The nurse, believing that Molly would best benefit by referral to one of the spiritual leaders of the church, listed that need.

The next step in the plan was to set mutually acceptable goals (page 334). Because the needs were divided into physical, emotional and spiritual realms, the goals had to follow that pattern to address all aspects of the person and promote holistic healing. The goal for the physical realm was that Molly would demonstrate knowledge of the control and maintenance of hypertension as evidenced by blood pressure within normal parameters. The goal for the emotional realm was that Molly demonstrate increased involvement in the church's seniors group and congregational activities. The goal for the spiritual realm was that Molly would demonstrate fewer signs of spiritual distress, such as wanting to die or the fear of death.

The nurse got Molly's permission to refer her to the appropriate resources, assuring her that all information would be confidential within the referrals. After obtaining Molly's permission, the nurse planned the interventions within each of the congregational nursing roles.

She developed a teaching plan regarding blood pressure which was personalized and specific for Molly because of her reading deficit. The teaching plan would include a video on blood pressure, question/answer sessions and talking about strategies for control. Although this plan was designed around Molly's circumstances, the nurse opened that teaching program to the seniors group so that all could benefit, and so that Molly could begin to develop a support system within the church family.

Health counseling needs regarding blood pressure and its effects on the whole person, including the physical, emotional and spiritual aspects were included within the teaching but were also continued with follow-up meetings and blood pressure checks. Counseling was focused on maintenance of optimum wellness and prevention of associated blood pressure complications.

Referrals were made to Molly's physician to address her hypertension and to the church pastor to address the emotional and spiritual needs. Multi-disciplinary referrals provided Molly a greater possibility of meeting her goals and achieving her optimum wellness. Referrals were also made to senior citizen support groups, groups which provide emotional support and help for the bereaved and to the American Heart Association for further information or help regarding her blood pressure.

The nurse looked within the congregation to get help for Molly. Transportation seemed to be Molly's biggest advocacy need, so the nurse arranged for rides to and from appointments, the store, church services and functions. Seeking help from within the church strengthened Molly's support system and allowed the church members the opportunity to serve God by serving Molly.

Follow up and evaluation of Molly's care was concurrent with the interventions so that replanning could occur if necessary. The nurse recorded the times that she and Molly met or spoke regarding the issues addressed in the plan, success of

HOLISTIC CARE SUMMARY		
Nurse_____ Date _____ Update _____ **Personal**	**Objective-Subjective Holistic Needs Assessment**	**Follow Up (Evaluation)**
Name _____	(Specify Needs) **Physical**	Number of times met _____
Age _____ Birthdate _____	1. Teaching _____	Regarding _____
Life Event Dates (specify) _____	2. Counseling _____	Number of contacts from RN _____
	3. Referral _____	Regarding _____
	4. Advocacy _____	Success of referrals as evidenced by
Current Support Systems (specify) _____	5. Other _____	Client attendance _____
	Emotional	
	1. Teaching _____	Client statements _____
Preferred Learning Style _____	2. Counseling _____	Success of teaching/counseling as evidenced by
	3. Referral _____	Change in client behavior _____
	4. Advocacy _____	Client statements _____
Learning Strengths/Barriers _____	5. Other _____	Goals met or unmet _____
	Spiritual	
	1. Teaching _____	Replanning _____
Experiences with Learning _____	2. Counseling _____	
	3. Referral _____	Other _____
	4. Advocacy _____	
©Renae Schumann, 1996	5. Other _____	

referrals, success of teaching or counseling, and whether or not the physical, emotional and spiritual goals were being met. Molly's statements regarding her care included, "It is so good to be back with the family. I had forgotten how much good a loving heart can do when a person is sad. I love the people who are helping me, and I want to live long enough to help them if I can."

The plan, developed according to the Holistic Care Summary (HCS), was complete and comprehensive enough to meet Molly's needs and to help her regain her optimum level of wellness in the physical, emotional and spiritual realms. Whole-person or holistic planning and care as directed by the HCS helps to ensure that all the client's needs are met equally, and that none are forgotten. Nurses know that holistic healing of the person's body, mind and spirit is necessary for wellness, because if one of the aspects of the person is affected, then all are affected. Molly would have seen no reason to learn to manage her hypertension if she felt alone and was tired of living, so it was important that the whole person received care. Meeting her emotional and spiritual needs in conjunction with the physical disease aided Molly's healing process.

Exact record keeping allows for more organized care, better communication among caregivers and greater ease and effectiveness in program and project evaluation. Periodic review of client records can reveal congregational health needs and trends, strengths and weaknesses in care delivered, and need to revise the congregational nursing care practice.

HOLISTIC CARE STRATEGIES						
Goals		**Care Possibilities/Interventions**				
Stated Client Goals	**Actual Client Goals**	**Teaching**	**Counseling**	**Referral**	**Advocacy**	**Other**
Physical—	Physical—	Group	Regarding	Physical Needs	**Within Congregation**	**Physical—**
		Personal			Meals	
		Specific Strategies Topic Literature	Physical	Emotional	Transportation	
Emotional—	Emotional—				Assistance	**Emotional—**
		AV	Emotional	Spiritual	Visits	
		Question/Answer			Other	
Spiritual—	Spiritual—	Talking		Support Groups	**Within Community**	**Spiritual—**
		Other (specify)	Spiritual		Agencies	
				Community	Support Groups	
					Other options	

Through accurate documentation comes evidence of success in client care, as well as the need to replan some aspects of care. Clients who have had the benefit of congregational nursing care are able to contribute to the nurse's and the program's evaluation. If those clients are satisfied with the type of care received, they are more likely to offer favorable evaluations of the nurse and the congregational nursing program to the church leaders and the church members.

Nurse and program evaluations are more efficient and more accurate with documented evidence of effective care and successful programming. The nurse has no way of supporting claims of success in the congregational nursing program without providing documentation of services rendered. An undocumented program, even one that is successful, is less likely to receive funding or other forms of support and may even be tragically severed from congregational services in favor of other, seemingly more efficient, programs.

Based on the nursing process, holistic care principles and congregational nursing roles, the Holistic Care Summary is a complex tool designed to help the nurse plan and deliver organized, holistic care that falls within the parameters of congregational nursing practice. With this tool, the nurse can quickly determine the type of care that would best benefit the client. The HCS is flexible, in that it can be modified to fit the needs of any congregational nursing practice, or it can be used as it is to correspond to the nursing process.

Originally published in JCN, Spring, 1997

Contributing Authors

Betsy A. Anderson, RN, MS (as of original article)
is a clinical nurse specialist in pediatric nursing at the University of Minnesota Hospital and Clinics in Minneapolis. Her lectures on pain management in children have been abstracted in the *Journal of Pediatric Oncology Nursing.*
- *CNP* (as of 2002)
is a pediatric nurse practitioner and patient care director at the Diabetes Center at Children's Hospital & Clinics, St. Paul, Minnesota. She has twenty-two years of nursing experience: as a clinical nurse specialist, in staff development, in management and in academic roles. She has been a conference presenter, attends North Heights Lutheran Church and is on the advisory board of St. Joseph's Home for Children.

Frances D. Atkins, RN, MSN (as of original article)
is a PhD candidate at St. Louis University School of Nursing and a clinical nurse specialist in child and adolescent psychiatric and mental health. She works in three rural counties for the Missouri Valley Health Span Consortium, and has a lifelong commitment to her church community.
- *PhD* (as of 2002)
is a psychiatric/mental health clinical nurse specialist in private practice in rural Missouri, and is a volunteer nurse working at the congregational and international levels in the *Community of Christ.*

Maria T. Boario, RN, MSN (as of original article)
is manager of the Mercy Hospital Parish Nurses Program, Pittsburgh, Pennsylvania, and has worked for over twenty years in community health nursing, including with Navajo Indians in Arizona and Vietnamese refugees in California.

Pattie Boyes, RN, BScN, MEd (as of original article)
is an education instructor at Victoria General Hospital, Winnipeg, Manitoba, Canada. She was a graduate student when she set up parish nurse practices at Elmwood Church of the Nazarene and the Salvation

Army Hampton Community Citadel, and has experience in public health, geriatrics, missionary nursing and teaching health care aides. She plays flute on the worship team at New Hope Community Church of the Nazarene in Winnipeg.

Ramona Cass, RN, Ph.D. (as of 2002) 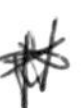
was founding editor of *Journal of Christian Nursing*. She is a United Methodist pastor, and earned her doctoral degree in Clinical Psychology from the Graduate School of Psychology at Fuller Seminary, Pasadena, California. She is currently a pastoral educator at St. Elizabeth's Medical Center, Boston, Massachusetts, and a psychologist in private practice.

Nancy J. Crigger, RN, PhD (as of original article)
is an assistant professor at the University of Central Florida in Orlando, has been on four mission trips to Honduras and one to Russia. She taught the adult Sunday-school class at her church for four years.

Marcia L. Denine, LPN (as of original article)
a nurse for 25 years, certified in long-term care, she is working on an RN through Regents College in New York, and taking pastoral counseling courses. She has published in *Journal of Geriatric Nursing* and *A Journal of Christian Healing* and attends Faith Community Church on Martha's Vineyard in Massachusetts.

Richard J. Fehring, RN, DNSc (as of original article)
is an assistant professor at Marquette University College of Nursing. He served as a captain in the US Army Nurse Corps, then earned his master's and doctoral degrees at the Catholic University of America.

Marilyn Frenn, RN, MSN (as of original article)
is an assistant professor at Marquette University College of Nursing and a doctoral student at the University of Wisconsin at Milwaukee. She is a member of the Wauwatosa Avenue United Methodist Church and a nurse volunteer in the Wellness Resource Center.

- ***PhD*** (as of 2002)
is an associate professor at Marquette University College of Nursing.

Lygia Holcomb, RN, DSN (as of original article)
is an assistant professor at the University of Central Florida in Orlando, a nurse educator and a family nurse practitioner who has presented widely on health promotion, primary care and nurse practitioner practice. She coordinates a nursing center in a poor area of Orlando and volunteers with the homeless.

Jean M. King, MS, RN (as of 2002)
is the University of Iowa College of Nursing Regional Faculty Coordinator of the RN-BSN Program at Iowa Lakes Community College, Emmetsburg, Iowa. Prior to her current University of Iowa appointment, she worked in acute care, public health and nursing education. She has also served as curriculum and evaluation consultant in parish nurse grant projects and in hospice program development.

Janet K. Kuhn, RN, EdD (as of original article)
recently retired after fourteen years as an assistant professor in the College of Nursing at Villanova University. She was active in promoting a paid parish nurse position at Bryn Mawr Presbyterian Church, Bryn Mawr, Pennsylvania.

Kamalini Kumar, RN, BSN, MA (as of original article)
is a doctoral student at the University of Iowa, Iowa City, and has taught in BSN programs for 25 years in India, Canada and the U.S. She does staff development and leadership training for continuing education for nurses and ancillary health personnel at Mercy Medical Center in Clinton. She has developed curriculum and taught Medical Careers and Human Reproductive Growth and Development in public schools.

Mary Ellen Lashley, RN, PhD (as of original article)
is an associate professor in the Department of Nursing at Towson University, Towson, Maryland, and a certified adult and gerontological nurse practitioner and parish nurse at Loch Raven Baptist Church in Towson.

(as of 2002)
is Director of Nursing Ministries at Loch Raven Baptist Church, Towson, Maryland, and a Board Certified Clinical Specialist in Community Health Nursing.

Patti Ludwig-Beymer, RN, PhD (as of original article)
is a clinical quality specialist for Advocate Health Care in Illinois, and has practiced in a variety of acute and community settings. She has written and spoken extensively on parish nursing and quality issues, and is active in her church's religious education, the Genesis Center of Health & Empowerment and local health fairs.
(as of 2002)
is Vice-President in medical education and research for Advocate Health Care in Illinois. She has practices in a variety of acute and community settings and has written and spoken extensively on parish nursing, quality issues, disease management and research. She volunteers for a regional dance company, in her church's religious education program, and is a member of ANA, Sigma Theta Tau and the Transcultural Nursing Society.

Karen H. Martens, RN, PhD (as of original article and 2002)
is a professor in the School of Nursing at Capital University, Columbus, Ohio. She has taught nursing for thirty years, guiding graduate students in their research. She volunteers in a program to feed the homeless and in the pre-Cana marriage preparation program. She attends the St. Thomas More Catholic Newman Center.

Lisa J. Mayhugh, RN, MSN (as of original article)
business analyst for Eclipsys Corporation and parish nurse coordinator at the Community Hospital, Springfield, Ohio, developed the parish nurse program and has been coordinator since 1996. She also developed the parish nurse program at her church, Central Christian, in Springfield.

Luberta (Skip) D. McDonald, RN, BSN, ThB (as of original article)
is a campus staff member of Nurses Christian Fellowship, serving the Southeast. She has experience in school nursing, home health, public

health, rehab, ophthalmology, post-partum, orthopedics and neurology. Besides an article in *JCN*, she has published in *Black Church Development* magazine. She is active in music and teaching at New Salem Baptist Church, Kennewas, Georgia.

Jeffrey J. McNeil, RN, MSN (as of original article)
a family nurse practitioner at Duke University Medical Center, served at a Christian family practice clinic in Power Springs, Georgia, as well as treating adolescent girls with STDs in a family planning clinic for several months. He was in youth ministry for seven years and leads the praise band at the Smyrna Church of the Nazarene. He previously spent two years in Adak, Alaska, providing health care to military families.
- *FNP-C* (as of 2002)
is a Nurse Practitioner at Duke University Medical Center and also serves as a bi-vocational pastor in the "Church of the Nazarene." He holds a Master's degree from Emory University, where he was named a Woodruff scholar. Jeff and his wife, Wanda, have two grown children.

Linda Miles, RN, MSN (as of original article)
a nursing instructor in the ADN program at Mid-Plains Community College in North Platte, Nebraska, continues as the parish nurse at her church, Vineyard Christian Fellowship, Curtis, Nebraska.

Susan L. Neff, RN (as of original article)
has a parish nurse distance learning program certificate and has served as a parish nurse for three years, serving two congregations in El Cajon, California.

Joyce E. Peterson, RN, BS (as of original article)
a school nurse for twenty years, is presently employed by Ballard Community Schools, Slater, Iowa, and serves as elementary school nurse for two centers with 650 students, kindergarten through sixth grade. She is in the early stages of a parish nurse program at Bethany Lutheran Church, Kelley, Iowa, where she is a member.

Susan A. Salladay, RN, PhD (as of original article)
is the director of the Center for Bioethics, William Jennings Bryan Memorial Hospital, Lincoln, Nebraska. She is coauthor of *Ethics in Mental Health Practice* and author of the "Ethical Problems" column in *Nursing '97*.

Renae Schumann, RN, MSN (as of original article)
director of congregational outreach for Memorial Healthcare System in Houston, Texas, was an assistant professor in nursing, Houston Baptist University. She is pursuing a PhD in nursing research at Texas Women's University.

Norma Singer, RN (as of original article and 2002)
retired after twenty-seven years as a staff nurse at Cook County Hospital in Chicago, has experience in pediatrics, operating room, orthopedics, and surgical and post-operative care. She is the author of two books and has written numerous articles in *JCN*, the *Chicago Tribune*, *Church Libraries* and *Nursing Spectrum*. She is involved in missions at Armitage Baptist Church and is active in Nurses Christian Fellowship. She is currently enrolled as a student at Northeastern Illinois University in Chicago in the Bachelor of Arts Degree Program.

Carol J. Smucker, RN, MA (as of original article)
a PhD candidate at St. Louis University School of Nursing, is a clinical nurse specialist in child and adolescent psychiatric and mental health. She works in three rural counties for the Missouri Valley Health Span Consortium. She has a lifelong commitment to her church community.

Phyllis Ann Solari-Twadell, RN, MPA, MSN (as of original article)
director of congregational health services and the International Parish Nurse Resource Center, Advocate Health Care, Park Ridge, Illinois, is a doctoral student at Loyola University in Chicago. She is the editor/author of *Parish Nursing: The Developing Practice* and editor of *Perspectives on Parish Nursing Practice*.

Lon Solomon, MA, ThM (as of original article)
a senior pastor/teacher at McLean Bible Church, McLean, Virginia, since 1980, he previously taught Old Testament studies at Capital Bible Seminary, Lanham, Maryland. Lon lives with his wife and three sons in Fairfax, Virginia.
(as of 2002)
Included in his innovative ministry is (1) Frontline, a targeted ministry for Generation X'ers, that has grown to more than 1,800 weekly participants in seven years, and (2) FOCUS and Soul Purpose, ministries to single adults aged 35 and over, serving 300 people each week. Lon and his wife have four children, including a special-needs daughter.

Betty Souther, RN, PhD (as of original article)
an associate professor at Houston Baptist University, Houston, Texas, is the director of the Center for Health Studies with four graduate programs in nursing and health administration. She has accompanied students on three trips to Mexico.

Sue Steen, RN, MS (as of original article)
an assistant professor of nursing at Bethel College, Arden Hills, Minnesota, has been in nursing education for ten years and teaches theoretical foundations, childbearing/childrearing, family nursing and leadership. She previously worked in pediatrics and obstetrics.

Jan Striepe, RN, MS (as of original article)
a consultant and the parish nurse project manager for Northwest Aging Association, Spencer, Iowa, is a parish nurse in her church. Jan is a speaker and author in the area of holistic health and parish nursing and has been involved in numerous related research projects.

Pamela Stuchlak, RN, MSN (as of original article)
is a certified Family Nurse Practitioner, who works in MetroHealth Medical Center's Emergency Department, Cleveland, Ohio. Pam attends the Independence Presbyterian Church and enjoys camping, hiking, photography, music, crafts and travel.
(as of 2002)
is a Family Nurse Practitioner with Singleton Health Services, L.L.C.

She is employed at NASA Glenn Research Center, Occupational Medicine Services, Cleveland, Ohio. Pam also *moonlights* in the emergency department of several hospitals.

Jack Sumner (as of 2002)
retired as Professor Emeritus from the University of South Dakota, and now living in San Carlos, Sonora, Mexico, a small community on the Sea of Cortez, a 6-1/2 hour drive south of Tucson, Arizona.

Linda L. Treloar, RN, MA (as of original article)
on the nursing faculty at Scottsdale Community College in Arizona, is a geriatric/adult nurse practitioner. She is a doctoral candidate at The Union Institute Graduate School studying disability and ethics in health and religion, and attends Scottsdale Bible Church.
- ***PhD*** (as of 2nd article)
on the nursing faculty at Scottsdale Community College in Arizona, is a gerontological nurse practitioner. She has personal experience as the parent of a twenty-six-year-old daughter with disabilities and did doctoral studies in ethics, disability and health care. She has previously published in *JCN* and regularly participates in JAF Ministries disability training.
- ***CS, NP-C*** (as of 2002)
a nursing educator in Scottsdale, where she teaches undergraduate and graduate nursing students, has bachelor and master degrees in nursing from the University of Iowa, is nationally certified as an adult and gerontological nurse practitioner following completion of a nurse practitioner program at the University of Arizona. In 1999, she completed a PhD in Disability Studies and Health Care Ethics, exploring spiritual experiences of adults and families affected by disabilities. Dr. Treloar is a frequent conference speaker/writer about integrating spirituality into health care, and disability and the role of the church. Publications include articles in the *Journal of Christian Nursing; Journal of Religion, Disability and Health; Journal of Transcultural Nursing; Journal of the American Academy of Nurse Practitioners;* and *Community College Review,* as well as chapters in *Bioengagement: Making A Christian Difference Through Bioethics Today* (Erdmans, 2000) and *Community Health Nursing: Promoting the Health of Aggregates* (Saunders, 2001).

Wendy Tuzik Micek, RN, DNSc (as of original article)
a clinical quality specialist at Advocate Health Care in Illinois, has done research, taught and written on quality and patient satisfaction for eight years. She is a trained clinical quality improvement facilitator, and volunteers at local health fairs.
(as of 2002)
is Director of special projects for Advocate Christ Medical Center in Illinois, has practiced in a variety of settings and roles, including acute care, operating room, ambulatory surgery and health services research. She has authored and co-authored publications, and presented at professional conferences in the areas of patient satisfaction, patient-centered care, nursing documentation languages and clinical process improvement. She is a member of Sigma Theta Tau, Midwest Nursing Research Society, Academy for Health Services Research, and Health Policy and American Association for the Advancement of Science.

Rosemarie A. Vandenbrink, RN, BScN (as of original article)
an active member of St. Mary's Roman Catholic Parish, West Lorne, Ontario, Canada, is a member of Sigma Theta Tau. As part of the University of Western Ontario's program for registered nurses, she participated in the development of parish nursing at Redeemer Lutheran Church, London, Ontario. With experience in surgery, medicine and geriatrics, she is in career transition from hospital nursing to a holistic nursing practice.

Cindy M. Welsh, RN, MBA (as of original article)
a clinical quality specialist at Advocate Health Care in Illinois, has experience as a staff nurse and clinical nurse manager and has participated on multidisciplinary process improvement teams. She has written and spoken on process improvement efforts in congestive heart failure and clinical quality improvement.
- ***BSN, MBA***(as of 2002)
degrees from Lewis University, and is the Administrator of Clinical Excellence at Advocate Health Care in Illinois, responsible for project leading development, implementation and evaluation of clinical excellence and patient safety initiatives in collaboration with interdisciplinary teams across the more than 200-site system. Management of Care across the continuum focusing on access, clinical care, prevention

and patient safety is key to this work. In her 19-year nursing career, she has worked in patient care delivery redesign, nursing management and clinical practice, has published articles in various nursing journals and is a member of Sigma Theta Tau International, Epsion Upsilon chapter.

Lynda Whitney Miller, RN, MSN (as of original article)
completed PhD degree requirements in August 1996. She has been a wellness educator for eight years and founded **Wellspring**, a wellness network in Canadian churches. Her article "Parish Nursing: Keeping Body & Soul Together" appeared in the January 1996 *Canadian Nurse.*
- RN, MSN, PhD (as of 2002)
an Adjunct Professor, Concordia University of Alberta, for whom she developed and taught a distance course in parish nursing based on her model. She serves as Parish Nurse of her local church and as Chair of the Parish Nursing Task Force of the Anglican Diocese of British Columbia. An author and international conference speaker, she is based in both Victoria, Canada, and Solvang, California.

Rita P. Wilson, RN, MSN (as of original article)
a medical case manager at Tacoma General Hospital, Tacoma, Washington, is a parish nurse at Word of Life Bible Fellowship (Church of God in Christ). She was a critical care nurse for eighteen years.
(as of 2002)
a Clinical Recruiter at MultiCare Health System, Tacoma, Washington, is a parish nurse at Roosevelt Height Church of God in Christ. She has been a critical care nurse and a case manager for twenty years.

Jean Wright-Elson, RN, MS (as of original article)
parish nurse at the 4,000-member First United Methodist Church, San Diego, California, served in the U.S. Air Force for twenty years and was an associate professor of nursing at the University of California in San Bernardino. She volunteers with the San Diego Hospice.
(as of 2002)
is no longer parish nurse for First United Methodist Church, Jean's concern is that no replacement had been hired as of publication of this book.

David Zersen, DMin (as of original article)
an ordained minister in the Lutheran Church, Missouri Synod, is the dean of the School of Adult and Continuing Education at Concordia University--Wisconsin.
- DMin, EdD (as of 2002)
has served as president of Concordia University, Austin, Texas for the past seven years. His most recent health-related project is a print/video study series funded by Wheatridge Ministries entitled "Wellness at Will."